Clinical Series No. 4

Report Writing

in the Field of

Communication Disorders:

A Handbook for Students

and Clinicians

Second Edition

by

Kenneth J. Knepflar

and

Annette A. May

Sponsored by the
National Student Speech Language
   Hearing Association
10801 Rockville Pike
Rockville, Maryland 20852

ISSN 0887-6584, ISBN 0-910329-61-3
Library of Congress catalog card number: 86-61408

NATIONAL STUDENT SPEECH LANGUAGE HEARING ASSOCIATION 1992

Regional Councilors

Region I
Tana DuBray
SUNY at Plattsburgh

Region II
Emily Crow
University of Pittsburgh

Region III
Jennifer MacDonald
Memphis State University

Region IV
Laura Harris
Murray State University

Region V
Kathleen Ralph
Northwestern University

Region VI
Katherine Spencer
University of Minnesota, Duluth

Region VII
Beth Bytnar
St. Louis University

Region VIII
Julie Weyrauch
University of Texas, Dallas

Region IX
Lori C. Ebert
Colorado State University

Region X
Jennifer Lamb
University of Nevada, Reno

Consultants

Sr. Charleen Bloom, Ph.D.
Chief Administrative and
Financial Officer
College of Saint Rose

Brian B. Shulman, Ph.D.
Convention Consultant
University of South Alabama

Leah C. Lorendo, Ph.D.
Consultant-at-Large
St. Louis Children's Hospital

Jack S. Damico, Ph.D.
Consultant-at-Large
University of Southwestern
Louisiana

Michael D. Smith, Ph.D.
Editorial Consultant
MGH Institute of Health Professions

National Student Speech Language Hearing Association
10801 Rockville Pike
Rockville, Maryland 20852
(301) 897-5700

Amy K. Harbison, NSSLHA Coordinator

Maria Michalczyk Palumbo, Production Editor

Table of Contents

CONTRIBUTORS

In order to make this handbook representative of a variety of work settings, a number of individuals were invited to serve as contributors. They provided sample reports and forms that were used as references in the preparation of the text. Some contributors took the time to write detailed explanations of their unique report writing methodologies, some of which are quoted in the handbook. Examples of many of the reports submitted by contributors are quoted throughout the text. Others appear in the appendices.

These speech-language pathologists contributed to the first edition of *Report Writing*. Some of them also provided new materials for this edition.

Nona Lee Barr, Ph.D.
Jefferson Parish Schools
Louisiana

H. Aubrey Feiwell, M.A.
Bloomfield Hills, Michigan

Donna R. Fox, Ph.D.
University of Houston
Houston, Texas

Jeannette K. Laguaite, Ph.D.
Professor Emeritus
Tulane University
New Orleans, Louisiana

Alan C. Nichols, Ph.D.
San Diego State University
San Diego, California

Irwin Lehrhoff, Ph.D.
Beverly Hills, California

James C. McNutt, Ph.D.
McGill University
Montreal, Quebec

Walter H. Moore, Jr., Ph.D.
Santa Ana, California

Gerald R. Moses, Ph.D.
U.S. Academy of Health Sciences
San Antonio, Texas

Francie L. Ross, M.A.
Atlanta Speech School
Atlanta, Georgia

Shirley J. Salmon, Ph.D.
Kansas City V.A. Medical Center
Kansas City, Missouri

The following individuals contributed to the second edition of this text:

Li-Rong Lilly Cheng, Ph.D.
San Diego State University
San Diego, California

Muriel F. Goldojarb, M.A.
Sepulveda V.A. Hospital
Sepulveda, California

Maureen M. Johnston, M.A.
Speech Pathology Services
Torrance, California

Patricia C. Lindamood, M.S.
Lindamood-Bell Learning Processes
San Luis Obispo, California

Lisa C. O'Connor, M.A.
California State University-L.A.
Los Angeles, California

Marguerite Orston, M.S.P.A.
Los Angeles, California

Glyndon D. Riley, Ph.D.
California State University
Fullerton, California

Jeanna Riley, Ph.D.
Riley's Speech And Language
    Institute
Santa Ana, California

Shirley Sparks, M.S.
Western Michigan University
Kalamazoo, Michigan

Helen Sherman-Wade, M.A.
Speech and Language Professional
    Services
Sherman Oaks, California

FOREWORD

During the past 12 years, students and professionals in the field of speech-language pathology and audiology have made extensive use of our fourth Clinical Series publication, *Report Writing*, authored by Kenneth Knepflar, Ph.D. Recognizing the value of this book, and responding to the number of requests for its publication, the members of the National Student Speech Language Hearing Association's Executive Council requested that Dr. Knepflar expand his original work, in order to meet the changing needs of our profession. Dr. Knepflar generously agreed to accept this challenge, and invited Dr. Annette May to assist him. We are grateful to both authors for their time and expertise in providing us with this contemporary edition.

When we reprinted the updated edition of *Report Writing* in 1991, we were sad to note that both authors died soon after the 1989 revision was published—Dr. Kenneth J. Knepflar in 1989 and Dr. Annette A. May in 1990. Because the material remains current, we feel that the reprinting stands as a continued tribute to their work.

Kenneth J. Knepflar, Director of the Communication Services Center in Pasadena, California, has been in private practice in speech-language pathology from 1961 to 1989. Prior to establishing his private practice, Dr. Knepflar's clinical experience included public schools, hospitals, and rehabilitation centers. An ASHA fellow, Dr. Knepflar had taught courses at several universities and lectured widely, particularly on the clinical management of stuttering and voice disorders. He was the author of numerous articles, book chapters, clinical materials, and cassette tapes.

Annette A. May, Ph.D., was Director of the Lincoln Center for Speech Pathology, Inc., in Pacific Palisades, California. Her facility was a rehabilitation agency, certified by the U.S. Department of Health and Human Services. Her previous clinical experience included 8½ years as Chief of Speech Pathology at a Veterans Administration Hospital. She had extensive experience as an off-campus clinical supervisor and CFY sponsor for graduate students. In addition to clinical teaching and administrative experience, Dr. May served on a number of community and national boards and committees. Her major areas of clinical expertise included language/learning disabilities and adult neurologic communication disorders.

Appreciation is also extended to Katharine G. Butler, Ph.D., for writing the Introduction to this handbook, and for so clearly highlighting the current areas of practice that this updated edition of *Report Writing* addresses.

Sr. Charleen Bloom, Ph.D.
Chief Administrative and Financial Officer

INTRODUCTION

It gave me considerable pleasure to provide an Introduction to the first edition of this handbook. I am even more pleased to be able to provide the Introduction to the second edition. The authors and their contributors have provided many new insights into that all-important activity of report writing, wherein one must make overt one's skills in diagnosis and assessment, in clarity of thinking and writing, and in being concurrently brief but comprehensive. If anything, over the past decade it has become even more crucial to be both explicit and highly skilled in the task of displaying your findings. As noted in the Introduction to the first edition, carefully honed and highly polished, the ability to transmit clinical activities and judgments will stand you in good stead all the days of your professional lives.

As someone who daily reads the reports prepared by graduate students in communication sciences and disorders, who prepares reports herself, and who receives innumerable communiques from neuropsychologists, audiologists, school psychologists, speech-language pathologists, reading specialists, and other special and general educators, I take particular pleasure in cogent remarks that define the parameters of the client's speech, language, or hearing problem. Although written reports, even the best of them, tend to be "decontextualized" (i.e., removed from the context of the moment of testing), writers who can provide some of the context by their remarks are to be prized. I would strongly second Drs. Knepflar's and May's comments that report writers should summarize vital information and interpretation of that information. They add that a mere listing of scores and other statistics is not enough. As the field of communication disorders has come to consider the evaluation of children and adults not only in the clinical setting, but in a number of other settings, descriptive information has come to be even more valued. Certainly, if one is to address concerns related to, say, pragmatic or semantic disorders, the social-communicative context is important and must be reflected in the written report.

Two new areas of assessment and intervention have come to the fore over the past decade: the evaluation of infants and toddlers (I-TODS), including observation of feeding patterns, prelinguistic behaviors, response to caregiver interactions, and so on; and the evaluation of individuals with communicative-cognitive impairments following traumatic brain injury (TBI). Such individuals, like those who are severely developmentally delayed, require extensive evaluation and intervention, utilizing a number of standardized and nonstandardized instruments. Accompanying these new areas of at-risk or neurologically damaged individuals is the continuing area of children and adults with language learning disabilities. As we have come to realize, while preschoolers spend their days learning language, school-age children spend their days using language to learn. Over the period of time between the first and second edition of this handbook, numerous research and clinical articles have reflected upon the interaction of the child's talk, the teacher's talk, and the text's talk. We have come to appreciate (and to evaluate and remediate) children who experience difficulties in the language of the classroom. And finally, today's clinicians-in-training need to take heed of the changing demographics in the United States, for they will need to develop skills in the assessment and intervention of not only white middle-class children, but also children from multi-ethnic populations who may or may not speak English, and are in the majority of many of the larger school districts.

The authors continue to highlight in this edition matters of ethics, privacy, and malpractice—matters that must be everyone's concern, whether as a student, a practitioner, or a supervisor. In addition, many states now have licensure requirements that clinicians should know, both to apply for licensure and to follow changes in licensure laws over time. The scope of one's practice may change over time with changes in national and state rules and regulations, third-party reimbursement policies, and a myriad of other regulatory or policy decisions. Now, more than ever, there is a need to remain current not only in conducting a practice in speech-language pathology, but in keeping abreast of health- and education-related issues.

Within the exemplars provided in this handbook, and the constructive as well as cautionary comments of the authors, the reader will find a tremendous array of suggestions for this most important endeavor: revealing yourself as a competent, analytic purveyor of information that is critical to the needs and aspirations of your client.

The National Student Speech Language Hearing Association is to be commended for sponsoring the second edition of this handbook. Dr. Kenneth Knepflar and Dr. Annette May provide you with information that can make report writing what it can and should be: rational, reasonable, and readable. In doing so they are to be congratulated!

As the edition goes into another printing, I wish to express my personal sense of loss on the premature deaths of Drs. Knepflar and May and acknowledge the loss to our professions. I knew them well; we will miss them both!

Katharine G. Butler, Ph.D.
Research Professor
Communication Sciences and Disorders
Syracuse University
Syracuse, New York

PREFACE

More than 12 years have passed since the first edition of *Report Writing in the Field of Communication Disorders* was published in 1976. During that time, our profession has experienced impressive growth. The membership of the American Speech-Language-Hearing Association now exceeds 60,000. Clinical services for children and adults with communication disorders have expanded significantly throughout the United States and other parts of the world. The percentage of speech-language pathologists and audiologists entering private practice has increased more rapidly than any other work setting. As our profession has expanded, the need for effective communication in the reports that represent us has also become more vital.

When the National Student Speech Language Hearing Association requested that this handbook be updated, we accepted the challenge, recognizing the need for a contemporary edition. Although some chapters of the original text have been only slightly changed, several sections have been modified and/or expanded significantly. A chapter on the applications of computers to report writing has been added. A number of important references have been added to the bibliography.

We wish to extend special thanks to those individuals who served as contributors to the second edition. Their unique areas of expertise have added significantly to the updating of the text. We also extend our gratitude to Linda Carmichael for her assistance in preparing the manuscript.

After the publication of the first edition of this handbook, NSSLHA sponsored the publication of a separate handbook, *Report Writing in Audiology* by Billings and Schmitz. To avoid duplication, therefore, most references to audiological reports have been deleted from this edition. For those who are primarily interested in audiology, we suggest that the two handbooks be used as companion texts.

We are pleased that students and professionals in the field of speech-language pathology have found the handbook useful. We are hopeful that this expanded, updated edition will continue to serve as a guide to those who wish to improve the quality of their professional writing.

Kenneth J. Knepflar, Ph.D.
Annette A. May, Ph.D.

Note. We are reprinting the preface as the late authors wrote it, for it expresses special thanks to those individuals who served as contributors to the second edition. The National Student Speech Language Hearing Association would like to add its thanks to those contributors and in addition acknowledge the outstanding work of the authors, Drs. Knepflar and May.

CHAPTER 1. A PHILOSOPHY OF REPORT WRITING

As specialists in the field of communication disorders it would seem particularly appropriate for us to be effective as communicators, in both oral and written language. Many of us have had some background in the subject area of public speaking, group discussion, and debate. Few of us, however, have taken courses in the area of technical or scientific writing. Nevertheless, we are expected to communicate our diagnostic and clinical findings to individuals representing virtually every aspect of the medical, paramedical, dental, and educational professions.

Opinions of us are often based upon the content, organization, and readability of our reports. Referrals are often made to us by individuals who have never met us personally and have never talked to us directly. Our letters and reports not only reflect upon our personal competence, but also on our profession as a whole.

It is the purpose of this handbook to provide basic information on report writing that will be sufficiently flexible to be of practical value to students and professionals alike, regardless of the nature of their training or type of job setting.

As we prepared the second edition of this handbook, we became increasingly aware that many members of our profession probably regard report writing as a necessary evil or as an unpleasant responsibility.

It is not surprising, therefore, that many of our reports are sketchy, poorly written, monotonous, and on some occasions overly technical and unclear. Our reports are needlessly long and cumbersome.

We believe that to write good reports, an important requirement is a more positive attitude concerning report writing. If we think negatively about report writing, our reports are likely to reflect negativism and the results may be misleading.

Most speech-language pathologists have had the experience of delaying the preparation of diagnostic reports. Even when detailed diagnostic information is available it is impossible to recall subtle nuances and information that may not be recalled if report writing is delayed. Emerick and Haynes (1986) make this statement:

> Put the clinical situation, the interview, testing methods, results and impressions in writing *as soon as possible*. Never trust a memory. Commit it to paper while facial characteristics and voice inflections can still be remembered. Make the report "alive" so that others can experience what occurred in time and place. The

1

raw data are of limited value to the clinician or other workers until they are assembled in a clear, precise, and orderly fashion. (p. 318)

Jerger (1962) states that contemporary scientists have to write in three different styles: (a) one for research proposals, (b) one for progress reports, and (c) another for the serious reporting of research in books and journals. He defines the special language for research proposals as follows:

"Proposalese" is a fairly stereotyped language system in which you must stress, by any means at your disposal, how it is that no one ever thought of this clever idea before in view of its far reaching theoretical import, as well as its significant implications for imminent clinical practice and rehabilitation. The secret is long words, complicated subordinate clause structures, and good old fashioned evasion. (p. 101)

Unfortunately, some of our diagnostic and clinical reports appear also to have been written in "proposalese."

We all recognize the importance of effective verbal communication, particularly in a clinician-client relationship. Murphy (1974), discussed the importance of communication to human existence, and aptly summarized a philosophy that can readily be applied to report writing:

To communicate fully means to be openly and honestly expressive and receptive in the presence of others with whom we wish to come into significant, authentic relationships. Between participants there must be something in common, a mutual problem, interest, or goal that has meaning for both or satisfies basic curiosity, need or fantasy. Life can be meaningful principally through what we have in common. This includes our modes of thought; it includes our language, it includes the speech of our language. (p. 39)

It also includes the writing of our language.

Our philosophy of report writing, then, includes something more than cold, barren scientific writing. Reports must not take on an air of extreme informality, but descriptions of human beings and of human behavior should not be reduced to mathematical terminology and form. In other words, test scores and quotients are often of much less importance than are the interpretations of these scores and the descriptions of the behaviors that were demonstrated during the testing situation. Too often, these vitally important segments of reports are reduced to a minimum or eliminated entirely. Without adequate interpretation and explanation, test scores should be taken "with a grain of salt."

We believe that the speech-language pathologist's role as a report writer should be one of summarization of vital information and the interpretation of that information. The approach, therefore, should be descriptive—not the mere listing of scores and other statistics.

In public speaking we learn the importance of audience analysis, in that good speeches are expressed with vocabulary and language that can be understood by listeners. Similarly, report writers should complete a "reader analysis" of their reports in an effort to insure that their reports will be understood and accepted by the persons for whom they are written.

Huber (1961), in his manual, *Report Writing in Psychology and Psychiatry*, states:

> If the student has some theoretical notions about personality and an outline for a report, he sometimes forgets the reader. If you overlook your reader, you are, besides preparing to write a poor report, missing out on the help the reader can give you. The first question to ask when beginning a report is: "What specifically does the reader want to know about the patient?" (p. 2)

The foregoing statement is directly applicable to the field of communicative disorders. A report based on diagnostic tests and/or clinical findings must be presented in language that is appropriate to the background and training of the reader.

Huber (1961), discussing the importance of "knowing" the reader of a report, says:

> Apart from discovering what happens to your report and obtaining new data, you can also learn how to write better reports by learning something about the reader himself. Do your best to find out something about him. Even the briefest answers to these questions will be helpful to you:
> What is his background?
> What professional terms and concepts can you use and be completely understood by him?
> What kind of language does he use?
> What does he weight heavily? (pp. 3, 4)

A copy of a report prepared for a child's physician would be generally inappropriate if sent to his teacher. This is true particularly if the report is filled with the "jargon" terms with which we often demonstrate the vastness of our scientific vocabularies.

We recommend any of the following three approaches be used to "tailor" reports to the needs of specific readers:

1. Prepare one complete report, including all vital information, eliminating as many technical "jargon" terms as possible. Send copies of this report to all professional persons who should receive it, with *accompanying cover letters*, which include interpretations of information contained in the report to those who receive it, (e.g., referring physician, school clinician, and classroom teacher).

2. Write separate reports to be sent to different recipients. This approach is particularly desirable when the main report contains highly personal background information concerning the patient's emotional and/or social situation. Such information should be sent *only* to the referring physician, psychologist, or agency, but *not* to a school or a classroom teacher.

3. Summarize report information in the form of a letter to the referring source. Other letters might be sent to additional professionals involved in the case. For example, a brief letter can be used to summarize the specific information about a particular child who stutters or concerning a child with a hearing loss; and copies of printed information outlining the procedures that a teacher might follow to help such children in the classroom setting can accompany the letter (see Appendix A).

CHAPTER 2. ETHICS OF REPORT WRITING

All speech-language pathologists and audiologists should be aware of the contents of the Code of Ethics of the American Speech-Language-Hearing Association (1987), the preamble of which begins with the statement:"The preservation of the highest standards of integrity and ethical principles is vital to the successful discharge of the responsibility of all members." (p. 59)

Report writing is one of the responsibilities that we must discharge in an ethical manner. Our reports must be truthful to the best of our abilities to make them so. We believe it is highly unlikely that any professional person would willfully present misleading information in a report. Most often, in our opinions, ethical standards are shaped by the kind of emotional adjustments that individuals have made, by the ways in which they handle their own problems, and by the insights they may have developed into their own needs and behaviors. In other words, we believe that most unethical conduct, in any profession, grows out of situations in which people have rationalized that they are right; and, therefore they believe that they are justified in their behavior.

In an ASHA convention paper, Knepflar (1973) made the following statement regarding professional ethics:

> One of the most dangerous "pitfalls" into which we may slip, as we pursue our professional careers as speech pathologists and audiologists, is the pitfall of *omnipotence*. In order to increase one's feelings of self esteem, these "omnipotent" individuals may come dangerously close to violating the ASHA Code of Ethics. They lose their objectivity and make statements that could suggest a *guarantee of results*, which the Code of Ethics states is unethical. (Knepflar, 1973)

Our Code of Ethics states that we must not exploit persons we serve professionally, that we must not accept individuals for treatment when benefit cannot reasonably be expected to accrue.

The sections of a report that must be written most carefully, from an ethical point of view, are those dealing with prognosis and recommendations. The following statement from a report of an 80-year-old stroke patient with global aphasia and severe dysarthria is subject to question:

Prognosis—Good. With a concentrated treatment program Mrs. Jones should make excellent progress in regaining basic communication skills.

Recommendations:
1. Mrs. Jones should receive speech and language training five times weekly.

4

2. Treatment should emphasize work to improve her receptive vocabulary and tongue, lip, and jaw exercises.

Clinicians who have worked with geriatric patients with severe neurologic impairment know that prognostic statements must be guarded and that concentrated treatment programs should be justified and outlined with more detail than the vague generalities made in the foregoing quotation.

Another ethical consideration pertaining to report writing concerns public relations. The ASHA Code of Ethics pertains to the responsibilities of members of the American Speech-Language-Hearing Association to other professional workers. It states that we should establish harmonious relations with members of other professions and endeavor to inform members of related professions of services provided by speech-language pathologists. What better way to accomplish this goal than through meaningful, well-written reports?

In recent conversation, a neurologist quoted a long, involved written report by a speech-language pathologist concerning a patient with aphasia. This report was replete with neurologic jargon that made it totally incomprehensible to us. When we admitted that we were unable to understand the report and asked him to explain it, he answered, "I can't explain it. It's a speech report. I called to see if you could explain it to me." We finally decided that the report contained the misuse of medical terminology; but even worse, it did not explain the patient's speech and language functioning, which is what the neurologist was seeking in the report, because it was written by a speech-language pathologist.

On another occasion a call from a physician expressed negative reactions to a letter from a speech-language pathologist, which concluded with a summary of his publications and professional vita. The purpose of reports and professional correspondence should not be to enhance one's image.

It is of great importance for each of us, not only in report writing, but in all of our professional activities, to be honest about what we know and what we do *not* know. A competent speech-language pathologist should not behave like a frustrated neurologist, laryngologist, or psychiatrist. Reports must convey our findings, but we must be willing to admit that we do not have all the answers. Huber (1961) makes this pertinent statement:

> To delete what you do not understand may do both the patient and your reader a disservice, since the data may be a crucial importance to the case. Data can have meaning to your reader because of his particular training in a special area or his additional knowledge of the patient, while you may have neither or these.

> Such information can be handled simply with a statement such as, 'While the examiner cannot interpret this behavior, the patient displayed . . .' Stating what you do not know is no reflection on your skill as a clinician; deleting your lack of knowledge is a reflection on your skill as a reporter. (p. 64)

Release of Information

In considering the professional ethics of report writing, Huber (1961) refers to "the dilemma of confidentiality." Just as psychological and psychiatric reports involve personal, intimate information, so do many reports in speech-language pathology and audiology. If placed in the wrong hands, or if not clearly understood by readers, reports can have profound negative effects on the lives of patients.

When a patient or the parent or spouse of a patient reveals personal information *in confidence*, it should never be included in a report without the written permission of the patient. This is usually accomplished by having a release form completed and signed, such as those presented in Appendix B. Release forms are available commercially, or can be made up and printed to meet the specific needs of a particular clinic or agency. A release form often is not customary when a factual report is sent out to the referring physician or agency. It is our opinion, however, that it is advisable for patients (or a child's parent or guardian) to sign a record release routinely, even in instances when the report is going only to the referral source.

When it is necessary for a clinician to request information from physicians and other professional persons whom the patient has seen in the past, the clinician should enclose a records release, signed by the patient (or a child's parent or guardian).

Huber (1961) recommends that psychologists and psychiatrists discuss with their patient what they are going to include in their reports. In this regard Huber states, "This procedure has even been found in some cases, to be therapeutic" (p. 85).

We often encourage patients to read reports and/or letters that we have written concerning them. Such experiences have stimulated discussions that have also resulted in the patient's development of insight concerning his or her problems. Another benefit has been in the patient's increased trust and confidence in us, because the patient has evidence that highly personal information, which was conveyed in confidence, has not been released.

The federal government has formalized some practices regarding release of information into regulations. Chief among these are the guidelines covering privacy and confidentiality. Privacy refers to the right of an individual to share or withhold his attitudes, behaviors, and beliefs from others. Confidentiality refers to the question of whether, and under what conditions, information about one person can be provided to another person. The codification of these concerns is found in the Privacy Act of 1974 (PL 93-579) requiring by law a patient's permission or that of a responsible party before a professional may share information with another professional or institution. This restriction applies equally to telephone conversations, memoranda, test protocols, or formal reports. In addition to the Privacy Act, a number of state laws and PL-142 mandate the terms under which patients and others such as parents, who have legitimate interests, may request to see records.

Malpractice Insurance

Just as physicians would not practice medicine without the protection of a malpractice insurance policy, no speech-language pathologist should perform professional services without such protection. A low premium group insurance plan is offered to American Speech-Language-Hearing Association members who hold the ASHA Certificate of Clinical Competence.

In training institutions students often are responsible for the writing of reports based upon evaluations they have completed. *Because in most instances students are not personally insured, reports that are prepared under their signatures should always be countersigned by a supervisor who is legally responsible.*

Similarly, reports written by (CFY) speech-language pathologists who have not yet completed the experience requirements for the Certificate of Clinical Competence must be countersigned by their clinical sponsor.

One of the contributors of this handbook, Fox, recommends that when a report has been prepared by a student, the following statement should appear at the end of the report below the signature of the student and above the signature of the supervisor:

> The above report was prepared by a graduate student in training in speech pathology (or in audiology) at (name of institution) and all information contained therein must be considered accordingly.

Huber (1961) again provides us with a message that we should read and read again if we expect to provide ethical professional services and prevent the necessity of having to use our malpractice insurance. He says:

> The endless question of how to handle confidential information can be solved to some degree by our constantly reminding ourselves of the limitations of our professional knowledge. We must also recognize that we cannot know or foresee all circumstances relating to a patient. Humility is some safeguard. But unfortunately the major safeguard lies in the morality and human decency of the report writer himself. (p. 85)

We suggest that many students and professionals too often neglect to refer to the ASHA Code of Ethics. We urge all readers of this handbook to familiarize themselves with this important document and to refer to it whenever sensitive ethical questions arise.

CHAPTER 3. ORGANIZATION OF DIAGNOSTIC REPORTS

Reports in the fields of speech-language pathology and audiology should be organized in a logical, systematic manner but with flexibility so that the specific aims of each report can be accomplished in the absence of superfluous information. It is equally important, however, that essential data not be eliminated. In this chapter, diagnostic reports, which ordinarily require the most complex responsibility for both speech-language pathologists and audiologists, will be discussed in detail. In Chapter 4 specific kinds of reports, including those that are routinely used in a variety of work settings, and those used for insurance purposes, will be discussed.

Speech-Language Pathology Report Format

A number of different organizational outlines have been followed successfully in the preparation of diagnostic speech-language pathology reports. We believe that a single organizational format may not be appropriate for all diagnostic reports. Variations in organization may vary in different work settings and may depend upon the type of communicative disorder being evaluated, on the procedures used and on the intended recipient.

The following organizational sequence is suggested as one acceptable format for diagnostic reports in speech-language pathology:

Patient's Name _____ Birthdate_____ Age_____
Address _____ Telephone_____
Date(s) of evaluation _____
Date of this report _____
Referral source _____
Diagnosis (Including Diagnostic Code Number)
Background Information:
Hearing Information:
Speech Mechanism Examination:
Articulation Evaluation:
Voice Evaluation:
Language Evaluation:
Fluency and Rate Evaluation:
Psychological Factors:
Clinical Impressions:
Recommendations: (Include treatment plan when appropriate)

If the patient does not require complete evaluative procedures in all of the areas listed (articulation, voice, language, fluency, and rate) a brief statement can be made in each of these categories, indicating that findings are negative. For example, if a patient has an articulation disorder and no other communication disorders, the evaluation might read as follows in the other areas:

Voice: During this interview the patients voice was normal in pitch, loudness, and quality with respect to age and sex.

Language: Oral and graphic receptive and expressive language skills were assessed informally and found to be within normal limits during this evaluation.

Fluency and Rate: At this time, all disfluencies were normal and rate variations were within normal limits.

It will be noted that all statements in the above quotation referred to the status of the patient *at the time of the evaluation.* This is important so that if a future change in the patient's condition were to occur, the report indicates that the status was normal at the time of the interview.

By including all aspects of speech and language functioning in the report, clinicians are less likely to omit important information. For example, persons who stutter often do not use their voices well, particularly during moments of stuttering; respiratory function during their communicative attempts is frequently inadequate. Similarly, individuals with language disorders also often have problems with fluency as they experience word-finding difficulties and problems in language formulation.

Many patients with neurologic impairments have difficulty in all of the areas mentioned. A sample diagnostic report concerning a patient with Parkinson's Disease exemplifies this point (see Appendix B). Other sample diagnostic reports also appear in Appendix B.

Identifying Information

At the top of the first page of every diagnostic report, essential details regarding the patient must be stated clearly and accurately. These "vital statistics" include the patient's name, address, telephone number, birthdate, age, date of the report, and the full name of the individual or agency referring the patient for the evaluation. The name and specific professional title of the evaluator should also be stated.

The appropriate diagnostic code number should also be included as part of the identifying information for diagnostic reports. Each medical and allied health treatable disorder has been assigned a Diagnostic Code Number. This is a classification system that permits easy computer access to information regarding treatment for any specific disorder. All governmental and third-party payer agencies require a Diagnostic Code for reimbursement.

A list of those codes that pertain to Speech-Language Treatment is in Appendix B of this volume. A complete presentation of diagnostic coding and procedure coding information for speech-language pathologists and audiologists has been provided by Flower (1984, p. 174–194).

The date of the report is very important, as are specific dates of any tests or examinations that are mentioned in the report. We have examined a number of reports in which dates have been omitted. Such omissions make it difficult for persons reading the report to understand the significance of the information included in relation to the patient's history.

Background Information

A complete case history is of vital importance to any diagnostic report in speech-language pathology and audiology. Huber (1961) discusses the fact that professional psychiatrists and psychologists frequently fail to take a complete case history. He says, "Our goal in diagnostics is to give meaningful information about a person, and one of our major sources of information is the history" (p. 11).

A number of good case history forms have been published. Emerick and Haynes (1986), Johnson, Darley, and Spriestersbach (1963), and Nation and Aram (1977) have developed case history forms which are useful in the diagnosis and evaluation of individuals with communication disorders. Specialized case history forms for young stutterers and laryngectomees appear in Appendix B.

For many years we have instructed our secretaries to make the following statement to persons requesting an appointment for an initial evaluation: "I will send you a case history form which we would like you to complete and bring with you at the time of your appointment with us." The case history form can then be reviewed prior to the interview, enabling the clinician to determine areas of the history that should receive special attention. It provides a guide to follow during the interview and some safeguard that pertinent case history information will not be overlooked.

Case history information that is totally irrelevant should not be included. Comments such as the following are probably not worthy of mention in reports because they could apply to most children:

"His room is very messy and he resists cleaning it up."

"He enjoys baseball and basketball."

"Her favorite T.V. program is Sesame Street."

However, pertinent factors that appear outside normal limits, such as prolonged high fevers, convulsions, a family history of communication disorders, and factors that indicate lack of stimulation or over-stimulation should be included.

A summary of previous treatment by speech-language-hearing professionals should be included as part of the Background Information section of a Diagnostic Report. In some instances a clinician may disagree with the previous diagnosis or treatment plan. It is important that these differing diagnostic opinions and treatment goals be summarized in the report. In such instances, it is particularly important that a report writer provide excellent documentation for any new specific findings or clinical judgments.

Some clinicians are overly concerned about offending other professionals by differing with their earlier findings. It is our obligation to our patients to have the courage to report our diagnostic findings objectively and completely, whether or not they are in conflict with those of another professional.

Hearing Information

In a report that is primarily related to a speech and/or language problems, at least a pure tone audiometric screening is essential. If audiometric test procedures have not been conducted, or if audiometric procedures have been conducted by someone else, or if it was not possible to condition the patient to respond, such information should be included in the diagnostic report. Whatever the circumstances, a statement regarding hearing *must* be included.

Speech Mechanism Examination

Many books concerning diagnostic procedures, including Johnson, Darley, and Spriestersbach (1963, Chapter 5), Emerick and Haynes (1986), Nation and Aram (1977), have presented complete examination outlines. It is not our purpose to reiterate such information familiar to all speech-language pathologists. However, we believe the important point that needs to be stressed is that too little information concerning the speech mechanism examination is included in many diagnostic reports by speech-language pathologists. Some of the diagnostic reports we examined in preparation for the writing of this handbook made no mention of the physical structures involved in speaking. It is not uncommon for speech-language pathologists to discover an organic problem or structural difference that has been overlooked by other specialists. Most notable among these factors is a congenitally shortened frenulum restricting tongue tip elevation, retraction, and protrusion. We recommend that a complete speech mechanism examination be included in the evaluation of every individual with a communication disorder and that all significant findings be reported in the diagnostic report.

Articulation

Many acceptable articulation tests and tests of phonological process analysis are available. The important point is that the name of the test used should be included in the report and the results of the articulation testing be explained in language that is readily understandable to readers of the report. Usually enclosing a copy of an articulation test is meaningless without an interpretation of the test data. A description of the patient's speech articulation should be made according to the nature of the articulation test procedure. That is, the interpretation and analysis of the test data should be reported consistent with the theoretical construct related to the particular test procedure. Therefore, results might be reported consistent with the theoretical construct related to the particular test procedure. Therefore results might be reported according to distinctive feature errors, or according to phonological rules, or in the traditional manner according to phonemic errors, in which case the defective sounds should be listed and the types of errors (omissions, distortions, substitutions) should be specified. The diagnostic implications should be stated. The following is an example of a traditional approach to articulation. The summary is clear and to the point:

> John's articulation development is considerably below normal limits for his age. The only consonants that are consistently produced correctly are the p, b, and m, which are among the first sounds expected to appear in a child's speech. Even these sounds are often omitted in the final positions in words.
>
> The most severe distortions and omissions occur on the consonants representing the voiceless sounds /t/, /k/, /f/, /ʃ/ (sh), /tʃ/ (ch), /s/, and /θ/ (th). John's hearing loss appears to be the only significant cause of his delayed articulation development.

Voice

We believe that voice problems constitute the most overlooked area in the diagnosis of communication disorders and that most training programs for speech-language pathologists are weaker in the area of voice than any other aspect of the field of communication disorders. Many clinicians do not use their voices well. It is possible that such individuals find it difficult to recognize, diagnose, and treat voice disorders. Our standards for normality with respect to voice are probably more broad and undefined than in any other aspect of communication functioning. Therefore, teachers and clinicians frequently fail to recognize the symptoms of vocal pathologies, unless they are extremely severe. In other words, so many people "play their vocal instruments" poorly that very few substandard voices call attention to themselves or interfere with communication.

We have made the preceding statements in the hope that more clinicians may begin to listen and observe vocal symptoms more closely in carrying out speech and language evaluations. We hope many clinicians will begin to report the mild and moderate vocal variations that, in our opinions, occur much more frequently than they are reported. Ask yourself these questions during the voice analysis process:

Is the voice "thin," weak, unstable? Is there huskiness or hoarseness that could be caused by vocal abuse? Is the voice produced with more than a normal amount of effort? (Is there movement of neck muscles and unusual movement of the thyroid cartilage?) Is the voice nasal or denasal to an extent that articulation is distorted? Is the vocal pitch generally too low or too high for the "instrument" to function comfortably? (Is there a significant difference between habitual pitch and optimum pitch?)

Specific information regarding maximum phonation time and the individual's vocal pitch range should also be included. If the patient's major problem is in the area of voice, many diagnostic procedures will be required, which are not described in detail here. In such cases, it is important that speech-language pathologists have all medical diagnostic information available at the time of the evaluation. If a patient with a voice disorder is evaluated prior to seeing a laryngologist, it is vital that a medical report regarding possible vocal pathologies be received before the diagnostic report is written.

We suggest that comments regarding vocal behavior should be included in all diagnostic speech-language pathology reports. We have evaluated several children who were referred because of delayed language development, an articulation disorder, or stuttering, who were found also to have a voice disorder. It is not uncommon, for example, that a child who stutters also has vocal nodules or a child with an articulation disorder also has velo-pharyngeal insufficiency.

The following statement appeared in the "voice" section of a report concerning a child whose major problem was stuttering:

> Tim's voice quality is consistently husky. Following moments of tense silence, which precede many of his stuttered words, he initiates phonation with a hard glottal attack. His release of air during stuttering is accompanied by extreme upward movement of the thyroid cartilage. His respiratory habits during both fluency and stuttering involve predominately upper thoracic and clavicular breathing.

The report also included a recommendation that Tim be referred for a laryngeal examination. The examination did in fact reveal the presence of vocal nodules.

Many adult stroke patients whose major problem is aphasia, apraxia, or dysarthria, demonstrate pathological voice symptoms. In such cases, a report, replete with the results of several tests for aphasia and a thorough articulation evaluation, is incomplete if a description of the patient's voice is not included.

Language

All diagnostic speech-language pathology reports should include a section on language. Even if the evaluation included little or no formal language testing, observations concerning linguistic behavior should be reported. The following statement from a report of a 6-year-old who stutters illustrates that the language section provided an important clue to both diagnosis and treatment.

> On Form A of the *Peabody Picture Vocabulary Test*, Dennis scored at the 9 year, 7 month level, demonstrating a vocabulary recognition level that is 3½ years above the chronological age (6 years, 1 month). His conversational speech is characterized by many compound and complex sentences, which he has difficulty formulating.

The clinical impressions section of the same report included this statement:

> Dennis has been unable to cope with the rapid, complex adult-level language with which he has been stimulated at home. While his language comprehension is advanced, his receptive skills, including auditory memory span, have not progressed as rapidly. Difficulty with expressive language appears to be a major factor in explaining the severity of his stuttering symptoms.

The recommendation section of Dennis' report included a statement of the need for family counseling to assist his parents and older siblings in their ability to decrease the length of their sentences, modify their speaking rate, and simplify their sentence structure when communicating with Dennis. If observations had not been made concerning language, Dennis probably would not have responded to treatment as well as he did.

When language symptoms make up a major part of a diagnostic report, it is necessary to report test information in a concise, easy to understand manner (see Chapter 6). Many physicians and other readers of speech-language pathology reports are not thoroughly familiar with tests such as the Porch Index of Communicative Ability, The Illinois Test of Psycholinguistic Abilities, The Minnesota Test for Differential Diagnosis of Aphasia, The Boston Diagnostic Aphasia Examination, or the Boehm Test of Basic Concepts. The purpose of each test should be described briefly and the meaning of test scores, scaled scores, and subtest score comparisons should be clarified. It is often helpful to quote specific responses made by patients to exemplify the scores and explanations.

For example, instead of saying, "Edith had difficulty repeating sentences of more than three words," the reader of your report would find this much more meaningful: Edith successfully repeated the sentence, "Please sit down." For the sentence, "Cotton grows in warm countries," her response was "Cotton grows . . . to the . . . hot . . ."

When language problems or unique linguistic features are observed, examples should be included in the written report. For example, one report of the language of a 5-year-old included this statement, which presents very little precise information regarding the child's expressive skills: Raymond does not make complete sentences. Many of his responses are "telegraphic." He omits many small words and he confuses the pronouns.

The following statement, including specific quotes from a language sample, is much more meaningful: Typical of Raymond's immature verbalizations are these statements that were made during the examination: "Him look at bird." "Bird fly up lamp." "Him no can get bird." "Him daddy help him."

When the report concerns an individual, whose primary disorder is in the area of language, it is important that specific information and scores attained from standardized tests be so identified. Data obtained by a language sampling approach should be reported, including a description of the technique used to elicit the response and an analysis of the content.

Language sampling is useful for describing syntactic forms and constructions. The report analysis should illustrate and describe language elicited in the sample. Because language sampling is not a standardized measurement technique, the findings should be identified in the report as being empirical in nature.

Helpful information to assist clinicians in obtaining, analyzing, and reporting language samples is included in a previous NSSLHA publication, *Clinical Oral Language Sampling* by Blackley, Musselwhite, and Rogister (1978).

Reports of language functioning are often both complex and confusing. In describing patients' language it is especially important that the written language of the clinician be concise and comprehensible to the reader.

You may believe, as many speech-language pathologists do, that a diagnostic report need not include a section on fluency and rate of speech if the patient has no stuttering or cluttering symptoms. Consistent with our belief that a speech and language evaluation should include observations of all aspects of a patient's communicative skills, we point out that little time or space is required to say. "His speaking fluency and rate are within normal limits." Statements to the effect that fluency is normal should be based on careful observations of a patient's verbal behavior. It is important that an attempt be made during each evaluation to get a sample of truly propositional speech involving description and/or the accounting of a personal experience. For example, short answers to the questions asked in an interview may not present a true picture of the person's fluency skills. It is advisable to ask yourself these questions during conversations with a patient: Does the patient use interjections (uh, well, er, you know) to excess? Are word and phrase repetitions prevalent? Are interruptions in the smooth flow of speech handled effortlessly or with some frustration? Does the patient frequently "grope" for words? Are frequent revisions and incomplete phrases present? Does the patient prolong consonants or vowels? (Prolongations are comparatively infrequent in normal speech.)

In describing the speech fluency of a person who stutters, it is important to write clearly and to avoid the use of "jargon." The following description from an evaluation report of a 25-year-old stutterer would be meaningless to many readers outside the profession of speech-language pathology:

> Ed exhibited both tonic and clonic blocks. His secondary reactions included facial tics and extreme muscle tension. Symptomatological variants included hard attacks and silent intervals.

The description above could have been more appropriately written in this way:

> Ed's symptoms include sound and syllable repetitions and tense moments of silence preceding moments of stuttering. Lip protrusions, head jerks, and eye blinks accompanied many of his communicative attempts.

Many reports regarding individuals with fluency disorders include little or no specific quantitative information. Two instruments, the Stuttering Prediction Instrument (1981) and the Stuttering Severity Instrument (1980), both authored by Riley are helpful in supplying such data. A sample test protocol using these instruments appears in Appendix B.

Psychological Factors

Because most speech-language pathologists are not licensed psychologists, statements should not be made that give the erroneous impression that a psychological and psychiatric diagnosis is being made. It is important to *quote* all pertinent available information from previous psychological tests or evaluations.

Observation of specific symptoms concerning psychological weaknesses such as nervous habits, symptoms of stress or frustration, distractability, inattentiveness, depression, hostility, or resistance should be described as clearly as possible. To avoid ethical and/or legal complications, speech-language pathologists and audiologists who are not licensed psychologists should *not attempt to interpret the causes of psychological symptoms and behaviors* that have been observed in evaluation or treatment sessions. It should be noted that some physicians are not pleased if speech-language pathologists use medical terms such as *symptoms of brain damage. Totally subjective impressions should be reserved for the Clinical Impressions Section of the diagnostic report.*

Speech-language pathologists frequently provide clinical services for individuals whose communicative disorder is influenced by emotional and social factors. In many instances, these circumstances have bearing on the treatment plan and/or the patient's prognosis. If, for example, a person (child or adult) experiences guilt, fear, shame, and/or avoidance of speaking situations, these attitudes and behaviors should be described in the report because speech-language clinicians must deal with these symptoms directly in the clinical situation. Direct quotations from the patient interview can be used to illustrate these circumstances.

In describing treatment approaches aimed at modifying attitudes and feelings of persons with speech, voice or language disorders, the term *communication counseling* can be used in the Recommendations section of the report. This term clarifies the fact that the counseling is related to the treatment of the communicative disorder and that the speech-language pathologist is not exceeding his/her professional limits.

Clinical Impressions

The Clinical Impressions section of every diagnostic report should be reserved for subjective statements that are based upon findings and observations that have been presented in the body of the report. Clinical "hunches" are often very accurate, particularly when offered by experienced clinicians. The important point is that such "hunches" be so labeled (see Chapter 6).

In the Clinical Impressions section, diagnostic findings can be summarized and explained. A concise statement of the patient's disorder, its severity, and causes should be stated. The following Clinical Impressions summary statements are typical:

James has moderately severe hypernasality and a mild articulation disorder. The major cause appears to be a velo-pharyngeal insufficiency (i.e., failure of the soft palate to make a closure against the posterior pharyngeal wall).

Kent has a mild receptive and expressive verbal language disorder. He has severe disabilities in reading and writing. His medical diagnosis of minimal brain dysfunction is supported by a history of seizures and an abnormal electroencephalogram.

Hal has complete aphonia (absence of voice) following total laryngectomy on May 27, 1975. Rudiments of an alaryngeal voice (esophageal speech) have been started by means of injection of air into the esophagus with plosive sounds.

Many report writers seem to avoid making a commitment in print regarding their "outlooks" with respect to anticipated clinical results and an estimate of the duration of treatment. Some reports include prognosis and recommendations together; others make prognostic statements in the Clinical Impressions section of the report; others use a separate heading labeled "Prognosis." Although its location in the report is probably relatively unimportant, its presence is vital if the report is to be considered complete. Our personal preference is to include prognostic statements in the Clinical Impressions section of the report, because in most instances prognoses are "educated guesses" that cannot be objectively validated.

Recommendations

This section should include statements concerning the type and extent of the recommended treatment program, including frequency and duration of projected treatment. Statements should also be made concerning referrals for additional testing, medical diagnosis, and educational placement. Also included should be recommendations for counseling that is advisable for the patient and/or the patient's family.

Flower (1984) suggests that we offer recommendations, not prescriptions. He states:

One of the most serious misapplications of a medical model to have plagued the delivery of speech-language pathology and audiology services is the assumption that evaluations lead logically to drafting specific prescriptions for management.

He further states:

Good clinical reports offer specific recommendations. But those recommendations should identify areas for further assessment, delineate important considerations for planning management, offer baseline descriptions of communicative behaviors, and suggest possible points of departure in therapy programs.

During the course of completing an evaluation, it frequently becomes apparent that additional information is needed. In such cases it may be necessary to refer the patient to professionals in other fields. To make appropriate referrals, it is vital that speech-language pathologists be acquainted with a variety of related medical and paramedical specialties. Professionals with whom speech-language pathologists most often interface include: physicians, psychologists, orthodontists, pedodontists, prosthodontists, teachers, clinicians, and audiologists. Among the physicians to whom members of our profession most often make referrals are those represented by the fields of otolaryngology, neurology, orthopedics, psychiatry, and pediatrics.

When discussing an outside referral with a patient it is necessary to obtain permission (release) from the patient to share written reports and to discuss the individual with an outside professional.

Concluding the Report

After all recommendations have been listed, every diagnostic report should include the signature of the examining speech-language pathologist or audiologist. Typed under the signature should be the name of the examiner, his degree, and his title (speech-language pathologist, audiologist), and/or academic rank, if appropriate, and the name of the agency or institution.

In states where a licensing law for speech-language pathologists and audiologists is in effect, we suggest that the license number and the area of specialization in which the license is granted also be included under the signature. This is particularly important when the report is being sent to an insurance company. For additional suggestions with regard to concluding reports prepared by students, see Chapter 2 of this handbook.

Alternative Organizational Formats

In some instances the detailed organizational format described in this chapter is not appropriate. For example, evaluation reports for most laryngectomized patients would not include a battery of language tests and in such cases, a simplified outline might be used. A sample evaluation report concerning a laryngectomee appears in Appendix B.

Many speech-language pathologists evaluate and treat children with language/learning disabilities. Lindamood, one of the contributors to this text, submitted a sample report of a Learning Ability Evaluation, which appears in Appendix B. Because this kind of report is highly specialized, it requires a completely different organizational structure.

In certain work settings, speech-language pathologists must adhere to specific guidelines for diagnostic reports, as required by the unique needs of their particular facility. One of the contributors to this handbook, Johnston, works in conjunction with a large Health Maintenance Organization (HMO). Johnston explains the report writing requirements of her HMO group in this statement: "The group encourages brevity in reports. I have been asked to shorten evaluations and notations." She is required to dictate reports which are transcribed by a transcription service. In these comparatively brief reports, speech-language pathologists follow an evaluation format that includes: Complaint, History, Summary, Impressions, Recommendations, and Goals. A sample HMO evaluation report following this format appears in Appendix B.

Diagnostic Report Letters

In Chapter 1, we suggested that in some instances speech-language pathologists prefer to summarize their diagnostic findings in the form of a letter to the referring agency or individual.

Reporting in letter form is particularly appropriate when a limited amount of information is to be conveyed and when the diagnostic information does not lend itself to the formal report format. Audiological reports, for example, are often presented in the form of a letter. Diagnostic information should be arranged in a logical sequence prior to composing the letter. Letters to teachers and physicians often provide the most appropriate format for presenting diagnostic information pertaining to individuals who stutter or have functional voice disorders (see Appendix B).

Audiologic Reports

As we stated in the Preface to this edition of *Report Writing*, specific references regarding the writing of Audiologic Reports is not within the scope of this handbook. Several sections, however, apply to both speech-language pathology and audiology. These include the chapters dealing with philosophy, ethics, style, semantics, and the legal aspects of report writing. For more detailed information regarding Audiologic Reports, readers are referred to another NSSLHA publication *Report Writing in Audiology* by Billings and Schmitz, (1980).

Consultation Reports

On some occasions, a speech-language pathologist may find it advisable to seek a second diagnostic opinion from another professional in the field of communication disorders. Consultation reports do not usually require a complete diagnostic evaluation, because the clinician requesting the consultation ordinarily would have already carried out a complete evaluation. A consultation is usually requested on occasions when a patient's progress is unsatisfactory or when the presenting symptoms are very unusual or complex. An acceptable consultation report should include a summary of background information, a statement of specific consultation requests, a description of the symptoms, clinical observations, and clinical impressions and recommendations which should respond specifically to the original consultation requests. A sample consultation report appears in Appendix B.

CHAPTER 4. SPECIALIZED REPORTS

Speech-language pathologists and audiologists frequently find it necessary to write reports for very specialized purposes. On some occasions special summary reports are required for continuation of insurance coverage. When Medicare and Medicaid (in California, Medi-Cal) services are provided, monthly summaries and daily progress notes are required. Special forms must be completed to fulfill the specialized needs of hospitals, clinics, rehabilitation centers, home health agencies, and the public schools.

This chapter will include discussions of a number of these specialized reports.

Referral Acknowledgments

A copy of an Initial Evaluation Report should be sent to the referral source(s) as soon as possible following the completion of the evaluation. The report should always be accompanied by a cover letter expressing appreciation for the referral and stating when treatment will begin. Flower (1984) emphasizes the importance of promptness in such matters. He says: "Continuity of client care and the maintenance of cordial relationships are best served when referrals are acknowledged promptly." (p. 103)

In instances when it is impossible to complete an Initial Evaluation Report promptly, (within 2 weeks) it is advisable to send a separate referral acknowledgment. Such acknowledgments inform the referral source that the patient has been seen for an initial visit, that the requested services will be provided and that a complete report will be forthcoming. This communication, usually in the form of a brief letter, should also include an expression of appreciation for the referral.

A sample form letter providing a general format for a referral acknowledgment appears in Appendix E.

Written Treatment Plans

Although treatment plans frequently form one section of evaluation reports, they may be written as separate entities. Treatment plans are required in most treatment centers because of the regulations imposed by governmental or accreditation agencies or third-party payers.

Written treatment plans are required by ASHA's Professional Services Board when considering a treatment program for accreditation.

These criterion for treatment plans have been listed by the ASHA Professional Services Board (1983):

A. Each client is assigned to a qualified speech-language pathologist or audiologist who assumes primary responsibility for the management of a client's program.

B. Long- and short-term treatment objectives are specified and based on the conclusions and recommendations of a diagnostic evaluation.

C. Treatment plans include statements of prognosis.

D. Treatment plans are reviewed and modified to reflect the changing needs of the client.

E. Treatment plans specify the types, frequency, and duration of speech-language pathology or audiology services.

F. Conferences are held with other service providers to review client progress, to develop further plans, and to maintain an integrated and coordinated program.

To meet certain criteria for quality assurance standards or third-party payment, speech-language pathologists are often required to submit a plan of treatment before initiation of speech-language services. Indeed, such planning can provide a road-map that ensures appropriate management throughout the entire course of treatment.

The Care Plan is drawn from evaluation results, which provide diagnostic and prognostic indicators. It is most relevant when prepared after the completion and review of the evaluation or re-evaluation report. Because the Care Plan may be the basis for approval or certification by a physician, the structure should be simple so that specific information is readily obtainable. Economy of wording is particularly important in preparing Care Plans. The basic information that must be included in a Care Plan is presented in this outline:

Patient's Name
Date of Plan
To: Dr. _____
Diagnosis:
Goals:
a. Short-term
b. Long-term
Treatment:
a. Frequency
b. Duration
c. Modalities
d. Activities
Signatures:
a. Place for speech-language pathologist's signature and date
b. Place for physician approval signature and date.

A sample Care Plan appears in Appendix A.

Progress Notes

Each clinician is likely to have a preferred personal method of writing daily progress notes. Often these notes are too sketchy and too abbreviated, and although they may be helpful reminders to a specific clinician in reviewing what has been accomplished from one session to another, they are seldom very meaningful to anyone else.

Whereas some experienced clinicians do not routinely chart detailed notes of each clinical session, periodic progress summaries are required in many work situations. In most hospitals, daily progress notes must be entered in each patient's chart by the speech-language pathologist. Such notes should contain sufficient specific information so that they can be read and understood by physicians, nurses, and aides who have dealings with the patients. Therefore, it is particularly important that such notes not be laden with professional jargon and abbreviations. Suggestions should be included in the progress notes or elsewhere in the medical chart regarding ways in which staff members can communicate with patients with severe speech and/or language impairments, who are generally unintelligible to an untrained listener.

Huber (1961, Chapter 4, pp. 49–59) presents an unusually complete discussion of problems pertaining to therapy progress notes in the professions of psychology and psychiatry. He states:

> Writing meaningful and helpful notes on a fifty minute therapy session is not an easy job. Some therapists avoid the complications by simply not taking any notes ... A few clinicians claim that recording of any kind distorts the therapeutic relationships; they say that what transpires in a session should take whatever form it takes in the mind of the therapist.
>
> My own point of view is that therapy notes serve an extremely important function. Primarily they are for the patient's welfare. For the therapist, notes provides an opportunity to review what has been transpiring and allow him the contrast opportunity to reformulate the case and its progress. It may even be that one of the reasons most therapy continues for such an extended period is that some therapists do not continually attempt to formulate what is going on, how the patient is faring, and what the therapist's feelings are. If therapists took the job of writing notes seriously, they might find they are not helping some patients and should shift them to other therapists. Therapists might also find that the study of carefully written progress notes may even aid in cutting down the treatment period. (pp. 50–51)

Speech-language pathologists often experience similar problems in note taking, particularly with patients whose treatment involves extensive counseling. Whether notes are taken during or after the clinical session, or both, is an individual matter, but the *need* for the progress notes is, in our opinions, universal.

Like so many matters of clinical judgment, the decision as to whether or not to take notes during a treatment session requires clinical sensitivity. Huber (1961) makes this apt statement:

> On occasion the therapist will feel that, at special times in a session, note taking is not advisable. This may be because of the extremely personal natures of what

is being said (e.g., a tearful and deeply felt account of a tragic incident) or because the patient is in a highly emotional or perhaps paranoid state. In some circumstances taking notes is about as sensitive a thing to do as taking notes at a funeral. (p. 51)

Flower (1984) emphasizes the importance of recording negative incidents as well as positive evidences of progress. He states, . . . progress notes are important as a legal record of ongoing services. They may also be important as a legal record of untoward occurrences or other potentially litigious situations. (p. 106)

Good progress notes will usually include the following:

1. Brief notes concerning specific clinical management techniques and materials used.
2. Interpretation of how the patient responded and statements regarding the patient's progress.
3. Suggestions or assignments given to the patient and, when appropriate, recommendations for the next session.

When specific home assignments have been given to a patient (i.e., a home exercise program for a patient with a voice disorder) it is often good procedure to make a carbon or photo copy of the assignment or recommendation for the patient's permanent clinical record. Sample progress notes appear in Appendix C.

Private Insurance Reports

In many instances the costs of speech-language pathology and audiology services are covered partially, or in some instances, entirely by individual or group medical insurance plans. There is vast variation with respect to such coverage among insurance companies and among plans offered by a single company.

It is extremely important that patients convey to speech-language pathologists and audiologists the specific wording of their policies before the necessary forms are completed and sent to insurance companies. Minor changes in the wording of a diagnostic statement can make the difference between acceptance and rejection of a claim by an insurance company.

For example, the explanation of services covered on one insurance policy reads as follows:

Restoratory or rehabilitory speech therapy by a qualified speech therapist, if required because of an illness other than a functional nervous disorder. If required because of a congenital anomaly, you must have had corrective surgery before the therapy.

It is apparent that coverage would be available for a child with a cleft palate who had had corrective surgery. It would also be available to a child with an articulation disorder, if a comparatively minor organic factor, such as a "tongue tie" had been a contributing cause. If, however, treatment was initiated *before* corrective surgery, no insurance coverage could be expected for the presurgical speech-language pathology services.

It is always advisable to attach a copy of a letter from the referring physician to each application for insurance claims. In such letters the physician should state the medical diagnosis and the need for speech-language pathology services. Copies of surgical reports, when pertinent, also can provide valuable supplementary information.

Many physicians, if not guided by the speech-language professional, provide referral letters so sketchy and general that insurance coverage may be denied, regardless of the accuracy of the speech-language report. Statements such as, "vocal nodules—please treat" written on a prescription form are not regarded positively by most insurance companies.

We frequently submit a "rough draft" of a referral letter to the physician to guide him/her in preparing a referral statement that will enhance the chance of a claim being accepted by an insurance company. For example, when an insurance policy will cover postsurgical benefits but may deny coverage when speech-language pathology services are recommended in lieu of surgery, the following statement in the physician's referral letter concerning a patient with vocal nodules would be very appropriate. "I recommend a program of voice therapy for Miss Brown to prevent the need for further surgery. Without vocal rehabilitation, the severity of the pathology would worsen, requiring surgery and post-surgical voice therapy."

It is particularly vital that private practitioners make it clear to patients and/or parents that *they* are personally responsible for the services rendered; that the insurance policy is between the patient and the insurance company. See Appendix D for a written statement regarding insurance which has been used to provide insurance information to patients at the time of their initial evaluations. If such an understanding is not reached, patients with limited financial resources, who assume their treatment will be covered by insurance, can run up a large debt before they are informed that coverage of their insurance claim has been rejected.

Another important point is that persons who make decisions regarding eligibility of insurance claims are sometimes poorly informed regarding the specialties of speech-language pathology and audiology.

In many instances, the insurance forms to be completed by "the physician" are medically oriented and do not provide space for an adequate explanation of the patient's communication disorder. Therefore, it is often important to attach a summary report that provides an *explanation* of the diagnosis in terms that can be easily understood. Fortunately, many insurance companies employ the services of certified speech-language pathologists and audiologists to consult on such matters.

On a number of occasions, claims have been rejected because of a lack of information or a misunderstanding of the information provided on the application. It is wise, in such instances, to resubmit the claim with a letter of explanation. Many claims rejected the first time have been reconsidered and accepted with more detailed supporting evidence and explanations.

In some instances we have received payment for services rendered to people whose policies exclude speech-language pathology services as covered benefits. The following statement was included in an appeal letter for a laryngectomee who was denied coverage for postlaryngectomy treatment services:

> As you know, after a diagnosis of squamous cell carcinoma of the larynx, Mr. Bork had radiation therapy and several surgical procedures, including a total laryngectomy, a radical neck dissection and surgery to close a post-operative pharyngocutaneous fistula. Because of medical complications following the removal of his larynx he was not ready for post-surgical speech rehabilitation services until November, 1987, at which time his surgeon, Richard B. Roberts, M.D., referred him to me.
>
> Although in the *Summary of Benefits* for Mr. Bork's insurance plan, speech therapy is listed as a limitation or exception, the plan does pay for "physical therapy upon referral by a physician". It also pays for artificial limbs and eyes. I assume that this plan would cover, not only the cost of an artificial limb, but the cost of the physical therapy that would be necessary for the patient to learn to walk with the prosthetic limb.
>
> Mr. Bork did not loose a limb; he lost his larynx. Just as your plan pays for an artificial limb, it covered the cost of Mr. Bork's "artificial larynx," a Servox electrolarynx. You have denied charges, however, for the specialized training he needs to use his electrolarynx satisfactorily and for the esophageal speech training required for him to communicate independently without the use of an artificial device.
>
> Esophageal speech training involves *physical exercises* involving training of the oral musculature to inject air into the upper esophagus and the training of the sling portion of the cricopharyngeous muscle to serve as a pseudoglottis, replacing the vocal cords as a vibrating source. The muscles of the esophagus are being brought under voluntary control to trap the air in the upper esophagus.
>
> The above described treatment procedures provide a kind of physical therapy for the muscles of the oral cavity, pharynx, and esophagus. It is my belief that the services being denied to Mr. Bork should rightfully be covered by the artificial limb and physical therapy clauses described in your *Summary of Benefits* pamphlet.

Less than a month after the above appeal letter was sent, the patient received notification that his esophageal speech training would be covered under his plan's physical therapy benefit.

In some instances it is advisable to request the support of the referring physician when filing an appeal. For example, on many occasions, strong statements from laryngologists have resulted in getting coverage for vocal rehabilitation services. The following statement was included in a physician's appeal letter:

> Without postsurgical speech-language services Ms. Jackson's vocal nodules would be likely to recur. Because her benefits covered the costs of her laryngeal surgery it would seem unwise to deny benefits for the only treatment that could prevent the necessity for additional surgical procedures.

Government Insurance Reports

In October, 1972 federal legislation was passed which mandated the establishment of Professional Standards Review Organizations (PSROs). These local organizations are required to review and evaluate health care services provided by Medicare, Medicaid, and Title V (Maternal and Child

Health) of the Social Security Act. A manual published by the American Speech and Hearing Association (1975) provides detailed information for speech-language pathologists and audiologists regarding PSROs. It is vital that all speech-language pathologists and audiologists, particularly those in private practice and those working in hospital settings, acquaint themselves with the details of this important manual.

The focus of the PSRO program is peer review, which is defined in the ASHA manual as, "The formal assessment by health care practitioners of the quality and efficiency of services ordered or provided by other members of their profession."

A special form, "Speech Pathology and Audiology Plan of Treatment" is explained in detail in the ASHA manual. A copy of this form, which was developed to create a system of uniform collection of data on speech-language pathology and audiology services, appears in Appendix D. Under the current system being utilized in California, this form is completed for each Medicare patient receiving services each month. The completed form must accompany the bill to the fiscal intermediary (Visiting Nurse Association, Skilled Nursing Facility, etc.) for speech-language pathology and/or audiology services.

Other special reports and forms have been developed by speech-language pathologists associated with home health agencies and federally funded regional projects to serve children with speech and hearing problems. Samples of such forms and reports also appear in Appendix E.

For Medicare reinbursement many compliances are required. This applies to both Part A (in-patient treatment) and Part B (out-patient treatment). The Part A status applies to patients in acute hospitals or, in special circumstances, to those in skilled nursing facilities. Part B applies to any authorized out-patient treatment: home visits, rehabilitation centers, and rehabilitation agencies. A procedure manual by Lehrhoff and Koroshec (1980) provides detailed information regarding reporting procedures for Medicare, Medicaid, and home health agencies.

The ASHA Health Insurance Manual (Downey et al., 1984) lists the conditions that Speech-Language Pathology services must meet in order to be furnished for Medicare beneficiaries.

1. The services must be rendered under a written plan of treatment established by a physician in consultation with a speech-language pathologist (if necessary) or by the speech-language pathologist providing such services, and the need for continued treatment must be recertified by the physician at 30-day intervals. (42 CFR 405.1717(b))
2. The services must be medically reasonable and necessary. For Part A, except for home health services, they must be directly and specifically related to the condition for which the patient was hospitalized, and must be reasonable and necessary to the treatment of that condition. The criteria of reasonable and necessary are met by the following conditions:
    a. The services are consistent with accepted standards of practice to be a specific and effective treatment.
    b. The services must be of such a complexity or the patient's condition must be such that the services required can be performed only by or under the supervision of a speech-language pathologist.

c. There must be an expectation that the patient's condition will improve significantly in a reasonable and generally predictable period of time, or the services must be necessary to establish an effective maintenance program.

d. The amount, frequency, and duration of the services must be reasonable under accepted standards of practice.

Although it is vital that clinical reporting be honest, it is also important that unnecessary negativity be avoided. Many Medicare and Medicaid recipients have been denied coverage for speech-language pathology treatment services because clinical reports and/or progress notes have inadvertently described patients' negative behaviors, weak responses or symptoms of resistance to treatment without reporting evidences of progress or encouragement.

Third-party payers, like most fiduciary entities, want some guarantee that they are receiving something of value for the money they expend. In the case of medical insurers this evidence of money wisely spent takes the form of records and reporting on the individual cases in question. These records and reports are routinely scrutinized by reviewers. The reviewers may be peers (ASHA certified speech-language pathologists) or they may be other health care professionals. In any case, they all look for the same basic assurances:

1. A diagnosis of a treatable deficiency or disorder.
2. A positive prognosis.
3. Accepted methods and procedures applied to treat the disorders including specific goals.
4. Measurements that indicate that progress and improvement is occurring and that realistic goals are being met.

Particularly when working with the Medicare system, it is essential that daily progress notes, initial reports and interim reports reflect these requirements. It is often necessary to spend several sessions building rapport with a patient who is intractable, disturbed, or discouraged by an interruption in communicative function. It takes time and patience to build trust and confidence; and motivating difficult patients is a valid goal in itself.

Throughout this handbook we have emphasized the importance of honesty and objectivity in clinical reporting. We have even stressed the fact that negative incidents should be recorded to avoid ethical and/or legal repercussions.

In some instances, however, detailed reporting of negative attitudes and resistant behaviors can result in immediate denial of benefits for patients who do have favorable prognoses. Therefore, we recommend caution when preparing progress notes or reports to be submitted with claims for private or government insurance benefits.

A positive tone is essential. Reviewers are not likely to "read between the lines" or synthesize information that is not clearly stated. If a speech-language pathologist records frustrations or persistent negative reactions by a patient, reimbursement is certain to be denied. Negative reporting can cost the patient an opportunity for rehabilitation services and a chance to regain communicative function.

If a claim is rejected at first reporting, there will be no opportunity to continue needed treatment, to break down resistance, or to establish rapport.

The following are examples of progress notes that resulted in a quick and unequivocal denial of payment:

3-3-87:   Patient in bed, minimally responsive to verbal stimuli. Attempted to elicit simple word responses to objects presented, but much of verbal output was "yes." Difficulty maintaining attention and frequent periods of feigning sleep.

3-4-87:   Patient sitting up in chair today. Immediately requested to go to the bathroom and then asked for a drink of water. However, when attempted to carry out an exercise in word recall—Answering "where" questions—patient closed her eyes and attempted to wave clinician away with her hand. It now appears that when patient is motivated she is able to produce the expressive language she needs.

3-6-87:   Patient in bed today responsive in terms of asking for water etc. However, when asked to produce automatic speech such as counting, days of the week, alphabet etc., patient waved clinician away and closed eyes.

3-9-87:   Patient relatively alert but uncooperative. She attended to therapist's conversation revolving around holiday that is upcoming, the foods used etc., but would not produce any conversational speech. At least she was receptive to stimulation, which is a positive step.

3-10-87:   Patient was sitting in bed today and again was responsive to clinician although unwilling to produce expressive language. Topic of patient's family was brought up, talking of her daughter and grandchildren, etc. But, she could not be stimulated.

Specialized Reports in the Schools

In her discussion of the school speech clinician as a professional person, Chapman (1969) emphasizes the need for mutual understanding between speech clinicians and members of other professions:

> Many clinicians in the past have recognized this need and have laid foundations for such interdisciplinary understanding and mutual acquaintances with services rendered, and yet there is pretty general agreement among these specialists that interdisciplinary communication is relatively poor, both with these individuals and ancillary services such as health departments and nursing services, and that each knows too little about what the others have to offer. (pp. 44–45)

Direct communication with teachers, school nurses, administrators, and professionals outside the school setting is invaluable. But effective report writing is equally essential. Fisher (1969) points up this fact:

> Records and reports play a significant role in public school speech and hearing programs. As specialists in communication we must communicate with others, keep others informed and prepare descriptive records of our work. One should have a good perspective of the need to develop and use efficient and effective

records and reports. A healthy attitude for fulfilling this responsibility is essential for quality records and reports. Clinicians should accept the challenge of this task with enthusiasm and a desire to do a professional job of record keeping and reporting. (p. 335)

Coordinated, clearly written reports, including case histories, daily progress notes, summary reports, and diagnostic information are of special importance in the public schools. This is true because of the likelihood that a number of different clinicians may work with the same child during his years of school attendance. A lack of clearly written reports often prevents the continuity of effective treatment services.

Black (1964) and Fisher (1969) present a vast assortment of record outlines, form letters, referral forms, and progress report outlines that are specifically suggested for use by public school speech clinicians.

Black emphasizes the point that records and reports in public school speech programs should be simple, accurate, and to the point, and that the tone should be both professional and friendly. She says, "Above all else, will this record, account, or letter contribute to better therapy for the child?" (p. 40)

It is important that reports of specific tests that are carried out by school speech and language specialists be written in meaningful language that can be fully understood by classroom teachers. Many reports of comprehensive tests such as the Illinois Test of Psycholinguistic Abilities and the Porch Index of Communicative Ability are so laden with jargon that they are of little value to teachers who have a major responsibility in the total habilitation programs for children with communication disorders. Sample test reports and letters to teachers are included in Appendix E.

Individualized Educational Plans (IEP)

The trio of initials (IEP) is well-known among those speech-language professionals who work in elementary and secondary school settings. The Individualized Educational Plan is a procedure by which children with special needs are assured that they will receive appropriate attention to their specific language/learning deficits. Those pupils in the schools, who are developmentally or educationally disabled and who require special placement, are evaluated according to a prescribed plan. School placement decisions and funding qualifications are dependent upon the IEP instrument.

It is important that IEP preparations contain information relative to:

A. Reason for referral for testing
B. History and background of the problem
C. Tests administered to determine:
   1. Phonology and expressive language
   2. Status of receptive vocabulary, auditory and visual response
   3. Social adaptability
D. Examiners' impressions
E. Recommendations for placement and special management

Weiss, Gordon, and Lillywhite (1987) present a more detailed sample format of an individualized educational program:

1. Current educational level of student (base line)
2. Long-term goals (for the entire school year)
3. Short-term goals (for every 2 or 3 months)
4. Special educational services needed (specific type of communicative disorder)
5. Beginning and ending dates of special educational services
6. Amount of time spent each week in special educational program
7. Justification for needing special educational program
8. List and specialization of persons responsible for implementing the individualized educational program
9. Evaluative procedures (administered twice a year) used for determining achievement of short-term and long-term goals
10. Recommendation regarding future status (to terminate or continue special educational services next year: include rationale)

An additional IEP format and an example of an IEP Functional Assessment report from a Head Start program are included in Appendix E.

Infant-Toddler Reports (I-Tods)

Another specialized area, for which some speech-language pathologists are responsible in their work settings, is that concerned with the evaluation of infants and very young children. Speech and language are difficult to assess in the first few months of life and few members of our profession have had the opportunity to develop expertise in this area of diagnostic report writing. One of the contributors to this handbook, Ms. Shirley Sparks, has provided a sample Infant and Family Diagnostic Report, which is included in Appendix E.

Reporting Assessment of Individuals With Limited English Proficiency (LEP)

Many speech-language pathologists find themselves faced with the task of assessing the speech and language of children, adolescents, and adults with limited English proficiency. Frequently speech-language professionals know very little about the client's native language and culture. Furthermore, they often are completely unprepared to test a client in his/her first language.

These problems appear to be particularly complex with regard to the testing of Asian/Pacific LEP populations. Another of the contributors to this handbook, Dr. Li-Rong Cheng has provided a sample report which exemplifies assessment information regarding a child with limited language proficiency in both Mandarin Chinese and English. This sample report also appears in Appendix E.

Checklist Reporting

Pannbacker (1975) discusses two basic types of reports: (a) narrative and (b) checklist. A checklist report is described as one "that has the advantage of providing information that is quickly interpreted by most report readers, depicting assets and deficits, and not requiring the services of a typist" (p. 370). Bangs and Rister (1969), King and Berger (1971), and others have developed such checklist reports. It is our opinion that a simple checklist report, in which diagnostic findings and recommendations are checked on a printed form, is often helpful as a *supplement* to a narrative report, but never as a substitute for a report that describes and explains in specific terms.

Supplementary Information Report

It is frequently necessary to record information pertaining to a patient's medical history or treatment program that does not fit appropriately into any established format. For example, medical information received from another professional by telephone should be clearly written and entered in the patient's case record. Important quotations or summaries of information revealed in a parent or family conference should also be reported as "supplementary information." Conversations that pertain to the patient, that have been discussed in a waiting room might also be considered in this category of reporting. A form that provides an efficient means for reporting these kinds of pertinent details is presented in Appendix E.

Discharge and Transfer Reports

When treatment services have been terminated, it is essential that a final summary report be prepared. Such a report should be written if treatment services have been completed, if treatment is to continue in another program or if the patient has discontinued treatment because of lack of funds, poor motivation, or dissatisfaction.

On a number of occasions we have requested information from a speech-language pathology treatment program in which a patient was seen previously. This information almost always has included an Evaluation Report and Progress Reports. Frequently, however, no meaningful Discharge Summary is included. When no Discharge Summary is available it is impossible to know the patient's clinical status at the time of discharge, how long he/she was seen for treatment, or the reason treatment was terminated. It is probable that Discharge Reports are less frequently prepared than most other types of clinical reporting.

Flower (1984) aptly outlines the ideal content of a Discharge Report. He states:

> Discharge and transfer summaries briefly recount the entire history of efforts to evaluate and treat a client's communicative disorder. They should begin with a concise summary of relevant services prior to the initiation of current services. Next, there should be a brief description of all services provided since admission to the current program, specifying the nature, goals, and extent of those services

and summarizing their apparent results. Finally, there should be recommendations for whatever continued services and follow-up are needed. (p. 108)

A copy of a final Discharge Report should be sent to the original referral
source. If the patient is to continue treatment in another clinical program,
a copy should go to that facility.

When third-party payers are involved, a summary of all previous speech-
language services must accompany requests for authorization of additional
services. Without Discharge Summaries from the previous clinical programs, such information may not be readily available.

If no Discharge Summary is prepared at the time a patient leaves
treatment, it may be necessary at a later date to attempt to write one when
requested by a specialist or agency who is currently providing professional
services to the patient. Under these circumstances, the report would have
to be composed by reviewing records located in inactive files concerning a
patient who has not been seen for a number of years. This is sometimes an
almost impossible task, particularly if the patient was seen by a staff
member who is no longer employed at the clinical facility. A sample
Discharge Summary appears in Appendix E.

Wilbur (1977) has discussed problems relating to the fact that no
standard record keeping format has been adapted in our profession. The
transfer of speech-language pathology records from one facility to another
would be greatly facilitated if there were more consistency in the formats
used and kinds of information reported. Wilbur's article describes the
Problem Oriented Medical Record (POMR), a system of organizing professional records which could be adapted by the professions concerned
with the diagnosis and treatment of communication disorders.

CHAPTER 5. COMPUTER APPLICATIONS IN REPORT WRITING

The computer revolution is upon us. Speech-language pathologists, many of whom are unsophisticated concerning microcomputers and their applications, cannot escape the fact that increasing numbers of references to the uses of computers are found in the professional literature, in the program offerings of our conventions and meetings, and as part of the equipment and materials available to us through publishers and suppliers.

Evidence that the use of computers is becoming more and more prevalent among professionals in our field is reported by Hyman (1986, 1987). In *The 1986–87 Omnibus Survey* Hyman (1987) reports the following:

> For the first time in the history of the profession, more than one-half of all speech-language pathologists and audiologists are using computers on the job. Nearly 54% of all survey participants indicated that they were using computers at least occasionally (i.e., at least once per month) in 1986. (p. 32)

Computers have great time saving potential in the area of clinical reporting. They can ease the burdens of clinical and administrative responsibilities for both professionals and students. They can be most useful in the area of report writing, particularly to students learning to write reports.

Data base programs are available for microcomputers that allow clinicians to select the information they want to store concerning their clients. Information can then be gathered quickly to be used for initial reports, progress assessments, and discharge summaries.

Record Storage

Computers can be used to assist in the storage of clinical records. Flower (1984) provides a comprehensive summary of the problems presented by a variety of systems of storing and retrieving records. With regard to computer-assisted records storage he states:

> Technology is now available to computerize all components of most clinical records systems. Computers can easily store numeric data, narrative descriptions, and even graphic representations such as test profiles and audiograms. The stored information can be retrieved immediately, either in segments or in its entirety, and displayed on a screen or printed out. Computer-stored records can even be transmitted immediately to any other facility that has the necessary hardware. (p. 168)

Rushakoff (1984) points out that although microcomputers can be helpful in maintaining client records, they also have certain limitations. He makes this statement:

> Even by using every possible precaution and backup, it's still possible to "lose" computer records. It is not advisable at this point for the clinician to replace standard paper records. Also, floppy disks tend to make it a bit unwieldy to maintain large records on a great number of clients. Hard disc drives, although much more expensive, are the most efficient component for maintaining client records. (p. 166)

Uses of the Word Processor

Students and professionals interested in applying computer technology to clinical reporting will find a chapter by Newton (1986) an important reference. In her discussion of computer software applications in private practice, she provides an overview of common standard software programs, useful features, user suggestions, and various applications in the private practice. Newton emphasizes the advantages of word processing in clinical reporting. Particularly helpful in this regard, is a listing of the specific features that are essential to those whose primary word processing needs are related to correspondence and patient reports. Also available are advanced software enhancements that check spelling, grammar, and syntax.

In addition to the uses of the computer in generating diagnostic and progress reports, Newton also summarizes a number of applications of the word processor in accomplishing the varied correspondence needs of professionals in our field. She states:

> The word processor does not take the place of those small yellow memo papers lightly stuck to various papers. It is very helpful, however, in producing the routine and not-so-routine correspondence of the private practice. Standard paragraphs can be carefully selected and arranged, or routine letters can be produced quickly from boilerplates. Form letters can be merged with selected names and addresses as cover letters for clinical reports, appointment letters, or letters requesting payment. Consider sending a boilerplate letter to new, potential referral sources, such as physicians or educators in your community, or a boilerplate letter to introduce yourself to agencies with which you may wish to contract for services. (p. 206)

The term, *boilerplate*, referred to in the previous quotation, is a standardized paragraph, which can be personalized by the computer through the insertion of demographic information (names, addresses, ages, etc.)

Setting up a Computerized Report Writing Program

Goldojarb, a contributor to this handbook, has submitted a list of suggestions for setting up a computerized report writing program for a clinic. Regarding Initial Evaluation Reports she recommends these steps:

1. Determine what kind of information and data is required by your clinic when evaluating specific types of speech and language impairments.

2. Set up outline headings for each kind of evaluation done in your clinic (aphasia, dysarthria, voice, stuttering, etc.) which will include all required information.
3. Two options for setting up the outline for the initial evaluation can be considered. In the first option, the outline may consist of the main headings with no subheadings listed. In the second option, subheadings are listed under the main headings to indicate the specific kinds of information to be included in the report. The first technique allows for more flexibility and individuality of writing style; the other offers more guidance and assurance that the required information will be included.

Goldojarb also discusses the advantages of the computer in preparing progress reports. She points out the fact that much information required in progress summaries carries over from report to report with changes and updates made as needed. She emphasizes the point that computer-generated progress reports assist clinicians to think in terms of continuity and measurable behavioral goals and of evaluating progress in these terms.

Goldojarb presents the following suggestions for programming the computer for clinical report writing:

The basic hardware required is a computer, one or two disc drives, and a printer. A number of word processing programs such as "Bank Street Writer" and "School Writer" are extremely "user-friendly" and quick to learn. A session or two going through their tutorials usually results in the novice becoming proficient in their use.

Using the word processing program you have selected, type in your report outline. Following program directions, save the outline on a blank disc using an identifying name: (i.e., "Initial Report," "Progress Summary," etc.). When you are ready to write your first report, again using program directions, call up the outline and begin writing your report under each of the headings. When you are finished, your report should be saved under the client's name. By using a different name when saving the report, the outline is not changed and remains intact.

Another of the contributors to this handbook, Orston, has developed the Communication Modality Summary (CMDS), a graphic computerized diagnostic summary of both standardized and nonstandardized test scores. This technique couples the graphing of test scores with computer technology. The CMDS graphs are accompanied by a narrative report. A sample CMDS overview sheet is included in Appendix B.

Public School Applications

Of particular interest to speech-language pathologists in the public schools is an article by Krueger (1985). She presents a system of computerized reporting designed and adopted by clinicians working a public school clinical speech program. This system generates due process paperwork, provides student reports and copies of Individualized Educational Plans (IEPs) and stores data for administrative and research purposes. The advantages of the computerized reporting system, discussed by the author, include the generation of more professional, easier to read reports, easier retrieval of data, and a saving of the time required for clinicians to complete paperwork and reports.

A study of factors that influence public school speech-language pathologists' acceptance and/or resistance to computer technology is reported by Houle (1988). In concluding her study, she makes a number of suggestions to enhance the acceptance of computer technology in our work environments, particularly in the public schools. She makes this observation:

> it is encumbent upon individual clinicians to upgrade their professional skills to meet the challenges of burgeoning technology. In addition, national, state and local professional associations must lobby for changes in educational policy at all levels to promote a work environment that will afford members access to technology and related training on behalf of students with communication disorders. (p. 426)

Sources of Additional Information

Whereas this chapter has been limited to a brief summary of information available regarding computer applications in report writing, we direct all students and clinicians to references that will provide in-depth information to those interested in expanding their familiarity with other computer applications in the field of communication disorders. Most notable among these is a text edited by Schwartz (1984) and two chapters by Newton (1986). The Schwartz text is a compendium of chapters by several authors presenting basic information concerning microcomputer hardware and software. Also included are clinical, research, instructional, and administrative computer applications to our profession.

Concluding the Schwartz text is a chapter by Chial (1984), who presents a glossary of more than 400 definitions of microcomputer terms, applied to communication sciences and disorders.

A variety of state-of-the-art software programs is currently available for use by speech-language pathologists to assist in generating reports, summarizing IEPs, and correspondence packages for use with clients, families, and administrators.

For further information concerning computer applications in our field, contact the American Speech-Language-Hearing Association's Committee on Educational Technology or the Computer Users in Speech and Hearing Group (CUSH) through the ASHA national office.

CHAPTER 6. WRITING STYLE

Training programs in the field of communication disorders typically emphasize the format and organization of clinical reports. Students seldom are taught the intricacies of writing style as it applies to report writing. Haynes and Hartman (1975) illustrate this point:

> It is our contention that there is a report writing style that we are attempting to instill in students. The problem is that we rarely teach the style, but expect the student to acquire it through trial and error. (p. 9)

It seems appropriate, therefore, to present a summary of some of the basic rules for writing style in report writing and to illustrate some of their dangers and limitations. Basic rules that should be considered are as follows:

1. Use specific language. Avoid ambiguous terms.

Klopfer (1960), Tallent (1988) and Flower (1984) explain and illustrate several styles of report writing that they believe are inadequate and potentially dangerous. Klopfer refers to "Barnum style" reports which he says contain universalities and ambiguities, "a lot of hoopla and very little substance" (p. 16). The following summary of a speech and hearing diagnosis illustrates a "Barnum" type report:

> Our tests indicate that Jim's language skills, particularly in reading and writing, are very limited, (four years below his age level). It is apparent that these symptoms indicate that he is functioning considerably below his capacity. It is probable that his language difficulties are caused by the insecurities he developed because of the poor interpersonal relationship he had with his first grade teacher.

The above quotation is not only "hoopla," it is largely inaccurate and unscientific. How can we say someone is "functioning below his capacity" when our diagnostic instruments did not measure his capacity? Are we entitled to say that a symptom is caused by insecurities, when our testing did not include a personality inventory and/or a battery of psychological tests? And are we, as speech-language pathologists, trained to identify a single cause of an emotional state? If we are not certified as psychologists and if our case history is limited to a form completed by a parent and a short parent interview, we think not. Also, note the phrase, "It is apparent that

37

these symptoms indicate that . . ." Why not say, "His symptoms show that
. . .," thus dispensing with some of the "hoopla?"

2. Use nontechnical language that can be understood by the reader. Define terms that may not be universally comprehended. Avoid jargon.

In writing a clinical report we often have a choice between using a
"jargon" word or giving a detailed explanation. According to English and
English (1958), *jargon* is a language peculiar to a particular trade, profession, or other group. Although it may require slightly more time and space,
the explanation method, rather than *jargon*, is usually the preferred choice.
Klopfer (1972) states:

> Many of the concepts utilized routinely by clinical psychologists are only
> seemingly complex and could just as well be translated into common predictive
> language easily communicated to anyone. (p. 2)

Huber (1961) makes this statement:

> Nothing takes the place of description and interpretation stated in simple and
> behavioral terms. Jargon should be used only if the words communicate clearly
> and meaningfully to the reader what the reporter wishes to say. (p. 75)

Speech-language pathologists frequently include in reports terms such
as *diadochokinesis*, without defining or explaining the meaning of the
word.

The following statement taken from a diagnostic report exemplifies this
idea:

> The patient exhibits limitations in his *diadochokinetic* ability, which indicates
> that a major cause of his articulation problem may relate to neuromuscular
> deficits and that his problem, therefore, can be best classified as *dysarthria*.

This statement should be criticized for the following reasons: The
sentence is unnecessarily long and complex; the terms *diadochokinetic
ability* and *dysarthria* should be defined or explained; and the reference to
neuromuscular deficits comes dangerously close to making a medical
diagnosis.

The information could have been written more effectively as follows:

> The patient has marked difficulty in producing rapid repetitions of the tongue,
> lips, and mandible in making rapid transitions from one articulatory posture to
> another. Mild fine-muscle incoordination is one of the causes of his articulation
> problem.

Moore (1969) gives this example of the overuse of "fancy words":

> The patient exhibited apparent partial paralysis of motor units of the superior
> sinistral fibres of the genioglossus resulting in insufficient lingual approximation
> of the palato-alveolar region. A condition of insufficient frenulum development
> was noted, producing not only sigmatic distortion but also obvious ankyloglossia.
> (p. 536)

Moore suggests that the preceding conspicuously jargon-laden passage could have been simplified by saying: "The patient was tongue-tied" (p. 536).

Frequently speech-language pathology and audiology reports are confusing because of the lack of consistency in the use of technical and clinical terminology. Laguaite, Riviere, and Fuller (1965) discuss problems pertaining to nomenclature and classification of communication disorders. They refer to Thompson (1961) whose system for classifying diseases and operations is generally accepted by the American Medical Association. Nicolosi, Harryman, and Kresheck (1983) provide an extensive glossary of terms used by speech-language pathologists and audiologists.

3. Use complete words which may be clearly understood by readers. Avoid abbreviations.

Jones (1971) says, "The forms and use of abbreviations vary so much in different fields that it is difficult to generalize about them" (p. 287). He summarizes several reasons for their use, but continues by stating that the case for not using abbreviations is stronger than the case for abbreviations. He lists the following disadvantages of abbreviations:

1. The reader may not be familiar with the abbreviation. If he is not, communication stops while he tries to translate the unfamiliar symbol.
2. The saving of the writer's time may be more than offset by the wasting of the reader's time.
3. The saving in space may be too slight to justify the time saved by the writer . . . (p. 287)

In the fields of speech-language pathology and audiology, abbreviations are used extensively. The letters C.P., for example, are often used as an abbreviation for cerebral palsy; but clinicians sometimes use C.P. as an abbreviation for cleft palate, and secretaries and nurses have been known to use c.p. as an abbreviation for chicken pox. Teachers often use c.p. in referring to the term *cut and paste.*

It is particularly important when writing reports to teachers that all technical terms be explained so that they understand as fully as possible the type of disorder, the severity, and how the problem will limit the child in the classroom.

In general, it is suggested that the use of abbreviations should be avoided in report writing, except when there is no question that the reader will understand their meaning.

4. Use a variety of language styles and word selections, according to the needs of the report. Avoid stereotypy.

Huber (1968) discusses pet ideas and stereotypy in report writing. He presents the example of a psychologist who mentions the level of "rigidity" of every patient. He says:

Rigidity is at best a vague concept; the use of such a concept is appropriate only when defined and when it is a notable symptom of the patient. Noting the *lack* of rigidity is like noting the lack of eleven fingers. (pp. 78–79)

With regard to stereotypy, Huber mentions that the reports of some people all sound alike. He suggests that the writers of reports should ask themselves these questions: Is this report essentially like the one I wrote yesterday and the day before that and the day before that? Could this report depict not only this patient, but all people as well? (p. 79)

Speech-language pathologists should be aware of the fact that frequently used phrases and stereotyped style and manner of presentation can be a serious problem. Terms such as *hyperactivity, short attention span, concrete behavior, rigidity,* and *perseveration,* which are used to describe the behavior of children and adults with neurologic impairments, are often used without definition, explanation, or illustration.

This statement from the report of a language evaluation of a 6-year-old boy exemplifies the problem of "pet phrases":

> Tom functioned poorly during the administration of the *Porch Index of Communicative Ability for Children.* His short attention span and hyperactivity often prevented him from listening to the test instructions. On reading subtests III, VII, and IX, he received only limited scores for his performance, partially because of his inattentiveness. He frequently perseverated.

In reading this report, a perceptive reader should ask several questions: How many tests were administered to Tom that day before he took his test? How short was his attention span? What were the possible reasons for the limited scores he received? What forms did his "hyperactivity" take? How many times did he leave the chair? On which subtests did he exhibit perseveration? What forms did the perseveration take?

It would have been more appropriate for this report writer to have said something like this:

> The Porch Index of Language Abilities for Children was administered after half an hour had been devoted to other tests. Because Tom's attention span diminished during this testing session, the Porch Index for Children should be readministered on another date. During the first five subtests he left his chair four times at intervals of 2 to 3 minutes.

> On Reading subtests III, VII, and IX, most of Tom's responses were delayed. Several times he required cuing before he could make a response. He made many reading errors, and there was evidence of perseveration, in that several times after making a correct response regarding one object, he repeated the same response for other objects.

Monotony often becomes a problem in report writing. If the frequent repetition of the same term or phrase causes writing to become sterile and monotonous, we suggest *Sisson's Word and Expression Locater* (1966). This easy-to-use reference is often of much more assistance than a regular dictionary or thesaurus.

5. Use specific, accurate, brief sentences. Avoid verbosity and needless words.

In her article, "Pathological Writing," Moore (1969) makes this statement:

The penalties for pathological writing are much the same as those for pathological speech, with one important addition. The written word remains after the oral
word is spent. The case for cleanliness, accuracy, and brevity in the use of
English is seldom greater than in clinical writing. Yet the profession which gives
primacy to oral communication sometimes fails miserably in written communication. (p. 535)

Most of us have had the experience of having to read a passage a number
of times in order to extract the writer's message. Sometimes we realize that
the task is impossible. In other instances, we find that a very simple short
sentence could replace what it took the writer a long paragraph to state.
The following passage from a student's diagnostic report of a language
evaluation of a 5-year-old boy exemplifies the problem:

When the examiner asked the mother if she interacts verbally with Richard she
appeared unable to understand the question, in that she answered: "Richard can
stay outside for the longest time and play with his dog," which made it seem as
though she was oblivious to her important role as chief interactor between
Richard and herself, in order to extract verbal productions from Richard.

It is not surprising that the mother's response was not adequate. If the
question had been, "Do you talk very much with Richard?" The response
might have been different. But if it appeared that the mother was still not
providing adequate verbal stimulation, the above statement could have
been reduced to:

Richard's mother was apparently unaware of the importance of her role in
providing stimulation for his language development.

We often do not realize that our sentences have become overly long and
complex. When you reread the rough draft of your reports *look for* such
unnecessary wordiness. Often a single confusing sentence can be broken
down into three or four concise readable statements.

Flower (1984) says that the first and most salient principle of good
reporting is conciseness, that the best clinical reports are the briefest ones.
He discusses the importance of brevity from the point of view of cost
effectiveness. He makes this pertinent observation:

Costs can be substantial if one reckons the clinician time spent in preparing
reports, the clerical time devoted to typing them, the time spent by professionals
who read them, the cost of entering and storing them in clinical files and of
retrieving them for future use, and finally, the cost of time expended by
professionals at some future date when they must locate specific information.
Ultimately, clients must pay these costs, or someone else must pay them in the
client's behalf. Therefore, responsible clinicians must continually inquire
whether the expensive words they set down in their reports are justified in terms
of their contributions to the client's care. (p. 111)

Flower (1984) also emphasizes the point that overlong and complex
reports can interfere in patient care. Relevant material can be lost in
verbose, wordy, irrelevant reports and thus, overlooked by busy physicians
and other professionals who are looking for factual information.

6. Convey a sincere, serious professional attitude in your writing. Avoid flippancy.

Being sincere and serious does not mean being overly scientific and technical. It simply means that we do not take a serious subject lightly. Descriptions of childrens' behavior are particularly likely to be described in informal, slang-laden terms. One student clinician's report stated:

> If he had been able, Bobby would have climbed the walls. He ran frantically from one corner of the room to another, opening closets, spilling boxes of cards and pulling pictures from the walls. He caused utter chaos and when he finally stopped for a few minutes, he made strange faces at himself in the mirror. All this time he was yelling and screaming like a wild animal with no recognizable words whatsoever.

Jerger (1962) says, "write it the way you would say it" (p. 101). However, if the preceding statement is an example of the way you would say it, we suggest that you modify your conversational style for a written report. Bobby's behavior could have been described more appropriately as follows:

> Bobby's hyperactivity took the form of aimless running from one part of the room to another as he explored his new environment. His verbalizations were limited to loud unintelligible noise-making.

In short, a professional report is no place for "cuteness" or needless inappropriate labeling.

7. Use complete verb forms and correct punctuation. Avoid contractions and hyphens.

This handbook will not spell out all of the rules regarding the use of punctuation, capitalization, hyphenation, the writing of numbers, grammar, or sentence structure. Jones (1971), Chapter 20, "Style in Scientific Writing," and Chapter 21, "Sentence Structure and Diction," are excellent references that review the basic rules for these technical details of writing style. Shertzer (1986) provides a particularly helpful summary of the rules of grammar and usage, including helpful tips on how to implement these rules.

A few obvious errors occur so frequently that they must be mentioned in this handbook. They include the use of contractions and hyphens. Huber (1961), discussing the problem of contractions says:

> Students often use contractions in an effort to make a report seem natural, the way a student would speak. The written word, however, produces a completely different effect from the same word when spoken. Contractions on paper are apt to appear strange to the reader, seem flippant, and both these reasons disturb the reader ... Contractions seem to some students to bring simplicity and lack of affectation. The fact is that they bring neither. A report is a formal statement, not a quote from a novel. Contractions should be used only when quoting the patient, if this is the way he speaks. (p. 80)

We would be inclined to add one other exception to Huber's statement concerning the use of contractions. We agree that they should never be used in formal reports other than in quotations, but in a letter (regarding a patient) to a professional person with whom you are acquainted, we believe that your writing may seem overly stuffy or pompous if you do not use contractions.

The following example from a report on a voice evaluation exemplifies the inappropriate use of contractions:

> At the time of the evaluation the patient stated that he *wasn't* having very much trouble with his voice. He also added that he *hadn't* noticed the problem during the past week. He *didn't* think it was worse when he was nervous.

Regarding the use of hyphens, Huber makes this statement: "Writers suffering from hyphenitis produce pages which look very much like a speckled hen" (p. 80). Hyphens, when used as a form of punctuation between parts of a sentence, can usually be replaced by a comma, semi-colon, or colon. Jones (1971) discusses rules for the use of hyphens. One important use is when two or more words are combined to form a unit modifier preceding the word or words modified. Otherwise, completely different meanings may be conveyed. Jones (1971) gives these examples: (p. 293)

A deep-green sea	a deep green sea
five-dollar bills	five dollar bills
12-hour intervals	12 hour intervals

The following quotation from a voice evaluation of a female college student demonstrates the incorrect use of hyphens:

> Dr. Gray had examined her larynx—no abnormalities were reported-the client said she did not recall that her voice changed during puberty—that at times she had been mistaken for a much younger girl on the telephone. Her medical history was negative-no frequent colds—no evidence of chronic hoarseness or voice loss-no excessive loud talking.

8. Use positive statements that show what testing or observations have revealed. Avoid qualifiers and noncommittal language.

Moore (1969) and Huber (1961) discuss some of these qualifiers or "leeches" of our written reports: *somewhat, probably, quite, sort of, kind of, may be, might be, appears to, seems to, it is believed, suggests, apparently.* Moore (1969) states:

> It may give the clinician courage to omit these if he remembers that the clinic report is not and does not purport to be a divine revelation of wisdom. It is not the pure truth. It is the truth according to a particular writer. Certainly it must not be over stated but neither should it be a timid collection of 'maybes' authored by a milquetoast. (p. 537)

The following summary of the test behavior of a deaf 8-year-old girl exemplifies the overly cautious, "milquetoast" approach to report writing:

> Linda *appears to have* adjusted rather easily to the testing situation. She did not *seem to* show resistance to her mother's leaving. She *appeared to be* a happy

little girl who laughed readily. She used *some* speech which *at times was quite* difficult to understand. She was *very* careful in making decisions and *seemed to* evaluate her responses before giving them. She *appeared to be rather* self confident and *extremely* cooperative throughout the testing session.

If all of the italicized words in the above quotation were eliminated, the statement would convey a quite different impression showing that the writer has confidence in his ability to make observations concerning the child's behavior.

Linda adjusted well to the testing situation. She showed no resistance to her mother's leaving. She was a happy child who laughed readily. She used language which sometimes was difficult to understand. She was careful in making decisions and evaluated her responses before giving them. She was self-confident and cooperative throughout the testing session.

It will be noted that the foregoing discussion of qualifiers and noncommittal language did *not* include the use of the term, *impressions.* There is an important place in clinical report writing for clinical impressions. The body of the report must be as objective as possible with positive statements that can be substantiated. Most reports, however, *should* contain a section clearly labeled *impressions,* which contains our diagnostic impressions or conclusions that are based upon clinical experience and expertise. Subjective comments and conclusions must be separated from objective findings in report writing.

9. Use personal pronouns when they are the natural way to make a clear statement. Avoid awkward circumlocutions.

Many reports in the field of communication disorders read as though words like *I, me,* and *you* were to be avoided at all cost. Referring to yourself throughout a report as "the examiner," "the tester," or in a research article as "the experimenter," sounds stilted and awkward. At times such avoidance of personal pronouns also makes the meaning confusing or misleading. Jerger (1962) makes the apt statement that:

nothing livens up dull material like *personal references.* Use them often. Especially use personal pronouns like I, me, you, she, they, etc. Don't use them to excess—the excessive repetition of anything makes dull reading—but don't be afraid to use them when they are clearly necessary in order to say a thing naturally. (pp. 102–103)

The following audiologic report contains a number of avoidances of personal pronouns. It also exemplifies several instances in which noncommital language is used unnecessarily and illustrates the improper repeated use of the word, *would.*

An *attempt was made* to determine Barbara's reaction to amplification by utilizing a hearing aid with an insert ear mold. Barbara *would* allow the *examiner* to hold the ear mold near her ear but *would* not tolerate the ear mold to be placed *by the examiner* into the ear canal. She *appeared* curious and was *seemingly* aware of the amplification produced by the hearing aid. This same type of curiosity and interest *was also observed* when *the examiner* placed a wrist watch near the child's ear. Since *this girl appears* to be aware of sounds of at least a moderate intensity level and because of her obvious rejection of the use of a hearing aid, amplification *is not recommended* at this time.

The above report becomes more readable and clearer when personal pronouns are used to refer to the examiner and to the child. It is further improved by changing the word, *would, to simple past tense.*

I attempted to determine Barbara's reaction to amplification by using a hearing aid with an insert ear mold. She allowed me to hold the ear mold near her ear but not to place it in her ear canal. She was curious and aware of the amplification produced by the hearing aid. She was similarly curious when I placed a wrist watch near her ear. I do not recommend amplification for Barbara at this time because she is aware of moderate intensity sounds and because she obviously rejects the use of a hearing aid.

The avoidance of the use of personal pronouns in referring to yourself, the writer of a report, often gives the distinct impression that you are not willing to take responsibility for the statements you are making regarding a patient. Statements like "it is not recommended that . . ." or "it was observed that . . ." or "it is believed that . . ." sounds like you are projecting the blame for the statement on someone else. If you do not have an adequate rationale for a statement so that you can comfortably say "I believe," "I recommend," "I observe," the best solution may be not to make the statement at all.

10. Use accurate, descriptive language that can be supported by fact. Avoid exaggeration and overstatement.

In her article pertaining to report writing, Moore (1969) says: The inexperienced clinician is vulnerable to this mistake [overstatement] and is poorly equipped to place superlatives into a frame of reference. (pp. 536–537)

Exaggeration and overstatement may cause negative reactions by professional people when they read a clinical report. Readers lose confidence in the judgment of the report writer when they detect the presence of sweeping generalizations and the unnecessary use of superlatives. The following phrases, taken from clinical reports illustrate this point:

Jack and Jim shared the same vocabulary of abbreviated words and were *perfectly* intelligible to each other.

Unrealistic expectations elicited *tremendous* anger-anxiety responses . . .

He was *extremely* attentive and *completely* cooperative during the testing situation.

He has *obviously* been a slow developer.

She was found to be a *very* exuberant child who *never* got tense.

He was *totally* unresponsive to auditory stimuli.

It should go without saying that when we are dealing with human behavior, words like *always, never, entirely,* and *completely* are generally inappropriate. It is also important in proofreading that we watch for expressions that would be more appropriate in a novel than in a clinical report.

11. Select the exact words you need to express a specific concept or idea. Avoid misusing words.

It is apparent that some report writers should refer to a dictionary more frequently. An otherwise intelligently written report can cause negative reactions from the reader if incorrect words are selected by the writer. A list of pairs and groups of words frequently confused in scientific writing is provided by Jones (1971). Some of these words that have been found incorrectly used in speech and hearing reports include:

ability, capacity	fewer, less
accept, except	good, well
adopt, adapt	healthful, healthy
affect, effect	imply, infer
among, between	in, into
amount, number	mutual, common
apt, liable, likely	per cent, percentage
attain, retain	practical, practicable
credible, creditable, credulous	principle, principal
explicit, implicit	unsolvable, insoluble
farther, further	valuable, valued

We suggest that this list contains only a few of the potential errors in word usage that confronts us in professional report writing. If you are insecure in this area, consult a dictionary frequently. Warn the secretary who types the final draft of your reports to watch for these kinds of errors.

12. Use active-verb construction whenever possible. Avoid passive-verb forms.

Many research articles and clinical reports in speech-language pathology and audiology are unnecessarily laden with the use of passive-verb forms. This writing style, although not grammatically incorrect, is awkward and difficult to read. Consider the following excerpt from a speech examination report:

> Jane was asked by the examiner to accompany him into the testing room. When she refused, it *was suggested* that her mother could accompany us for a few minutes. After a brief "adjustment period," Jane's mother *was able* to leave the room and test instructions *were given* to Jane and she cooperated as test items *were* administered.

This information could have easily been stated more clearly and concisely as follows:

Because of Jane's refusal to accompany me to the testing room, her mother joined us briefly. After her mother's departure, Jane cooperated during the administration of the tests.

Jerger (1962) presents several apt examples from *JSHD* and *JSHR* articles in which the passive voice is over-used. He refers to "an almost religious dedication to the use of passive-verb construction" (p. 102).

Strunk and White (1979) state that the active voice is more vigorous than the passive and that the habitual use of the active voice makes for forcible writing. They say:

> This is true not only in narrative principally concerned with action, but with writing of any kind. Many a tame sentence of description or exposition can be made lively and emphatic by substituting a transitive in the active voice for some such perfunctory expression as *there is* or *could be heard*. (p. 18)

The following excerpts from clinical reports exemplify the fact that direct use of active verb forms is not only more readable but usually shorter.

There were nasal emissions of air accompanying the production of many of his plosive and fricative consonant sounds.	He produced many of the consonant sounds with nasal emissions of air.
Erratic responses to many of the pure tone stimuli could be observed.	His responses to pure tone stimuli were erratic.
The reason that she finally came for the voice evaluation was that her voice problem had become much more severe during the past month.	Increasing severity of her voice problem during the past month resulted in her decision to seek help.

Summary

To summarize, the following should be avoided in report writing:

1. Ambiguous terms.
2. Jargon.
3. Abbreviations.
4. Stereotypy.
5. Verbosity and needless words.
6. Flippancy.
7. Contractions and hyphens.
8. Qualifiers and noncommittal language.
9. Awkward circumlocutions.
10. Exaggeration and overstatement.
11. Misusing words.
12. Passive-verb forms.

It is possible that some individuals, after reading all of the foregoing rules regarding writing styles, may respond to their responsibilities as report writers with even more anxiety than before reading this handbook.

We hope that such is not the case; but recognizing that writing may be difficult for some people, we believe that the suggestions to students provided by Emerick and Haynes (1986) may be of some assistance:

> Write on a daily basis. Each night—before retiring, for example—sit down and write a descriptive paragraph concerning something that happened that day. At first it may be halting and difficult; as in any new task, your writing "muscle" will be sore. Don't wait for an inspiration, for that magic moment when, suddenly, it will come to you. You go to it. At the end of a week, review the writing you have done—edit, revise, ask yourself what you meant by each word or phrase. The best way to learn to write, in our opinion, is to write.
>
> Get the message out and revise it later. A common error that some beginning writers make is to attempt to produce perfect writing in the initial draft. It doesn't matter how it looks at this point; you can always edit or have someone help you edit. When you meet barriers or mental blocks, jump over them and go on with the rest of the report. When you come back to it later, you will find that your mind has filled in the blank spots. (pp. 329–330)

We suggest that each of the 12 rules of writing style that have been summarized should be used by report writers in speech-language pathology. When in doubt, we hope that readers will refer to this handbook and other useful references that are listed in the bibliography.

CHAPTER 7. SEMANTIC FACTORS IN REPORT WRITING

"The language of science is the better part of the method of science" (p. 50). These words were written by Johnson (1952) in *People in Quandaries*. Johnson contributed, perhaps more than any other individual in the history of the professions of speech-language pathology and audiology, to our understanding of semantic concepts and their applications to our work.

In an article dealing with a semantic approach to clinical reporting in speech-language pathology, English and Lillywhite (1963) describe four levels of communication which provide an organized method of reporting and technique for structuring examination procedures. Their four levels, which are based upon a scientific orientation (as outlined by Johnson), are: observation, description, evaluation, and feeling (or hunch).

The *observation* level includes the oral examination, the administration of tests, the interviews, and the taking of a case history.

The *descriptive* level includes the process of putting the findings into words. English and Lillywhite point out:

> At this point the language of the clinician is most important. He consciously avoids being influenced or influencing others with his language structure. . . . He is constantly aware that 'emotive language' is out of order and he must depend upon unbiased description. (p. 648)

The *evaluational* level involves interpreting what has been observed. Judgments are made and hypotheses are formulated. It is at this level that the clinician reaches some "guarded" conclusions concerning his client.

The *feeling* level includes the process of verbalizing how we feel about what we have observed. It is at this stage of clinical reporting that an experienced clinician is able to list *impressions*, which cannot be developed into conclusions or hypotheses (see Chapter 3).

Most of what has been said about report writing in this handbook has been supported by the literature and/or by information that has been generally accepted by professional people in speech-language pathology, audiology, and other related professions. Every writer probably has certain points about which he or she has developed strong attitudes that have not been discussed in the literature or have not been widely accepted among authorities. We are not exceptions. Most of our "biases" are semantic in nature. We believe that we often use terms and word patterns, particularly in our written reports, that are easily misinterpreted by readers. We know what we mean, but inappropriate word choices may communicate something quite different.

The phrases "I feel that . . ." or "It is felt that . . ." are used much too frequently when we mean "I believe that . . ." "It is my belief that . . .," or "It is my opinion that . . ." The information that we are attempting to convey in a report should be as objective and factual as possible. The statement, "I feel that . . ." detracts from the objectivity of the report and removes some of the authority from what we say. "I feel that" should be reserved for the *Clinical Impressions* section of a report.

We join many other speech-language pathologists in encouraging the elimination of the terms, *therapist* and *therapy* in referring to ourselves and the services we perform. This is particularly important with respect to report writing. Unlike physical therapy and occupational therapy, the execution of speech-language pathology and audiology services does not ordinarily depend upon medical prescription. We perform our own diagnostic and evaluative services and determine our own treatment plans. It is vital that we not place ourselves in a position where our services and fees are incorrectly classified and limited.

An exception to the aforementioned statement that speech-language pathologists do not depend upon medical prescriptions exists in the case of certified rehabilitation agencies. All rehabilitation agency patients must be physician referred. Treatment plans must be signed by the referring physician and recertified every 30 days.

It will be observed that throughout the text of this handbook, persons with communication disorders have been referred to as *patients*, a term that we use almost uniformly in our work settings. We are aware that many students in our field are trained to use the word *clients*, because professional speech-language pathologists and audiologists should not imply that they are physicians, and persons with communication disorders are not usually physically ill. We believe that the choice of terms in this regard is entirely dependent upon the semantic requirements of each professional work setting.

Those who work in medical schools and clinics, hospitals, skilled nursing facilities, and in most private-practice settings usually make use of the term *patients*. Persons who are employed in mental health clinics, community speech and hearing centers, and in university training centers usually use the term *clients*. Those who are employed by private and public schools often use the term *students*. We believe that this particular semantic choice must be left to each individual.

When we refer to our patients or clients it is extremely important that we emphasize the fact that they are *people*. We refrain from labeling people by the names of their problems. If our oral public presentations, our publications, and our reports consistently followed this rule, we would improve attitudes toward people with communication disorders and the services we perform for them. We suggest that we refrain from terms such as *cleft palate child, C.P. child, M.R. child,* or *aphasic adult.* The phrases, "a child who has a cleft palate," "a child with cerebral palsy," "a child with intellectual deficits," or "an adult with aphasia" are preferable. We thus emphasize the fact that primarily they are people, and secondarily they have a problem.

In referring to "the moment of stuttering" in reports dealing with those who stutter, we suggest refraining from using the old, reliable term, *block*. The word *block* carries a connotation of some sort of impenetrable barrier, or of a physical or neurological blockage, or even of the much overused term *mental block*. It is just as easy to use *the moment of stuttering* or *the symptom*, terms that do not carry a negative or misleading semantic value.

Other words which we believe should be used less frequently are the terms *handicap, defect, impediment*. Unfortunately, to many people these words carry the connotation of a physically crippling disorder or of an irreversible disease or anomaly. Often when we first see a person who stutters, a child with an articulation disorder, a child with a cleft palate, an adult with aphasia, or a person with a hearing problem, that individual *is* handicapped. That is, he or she cannot function academically or vocationally in a hearing, speaking world. Hopefully our clinical services will aid our clients to function more adequately. Why then, from our first contact with patients, should we not refer to their symptoms or problems or disorders, rather than handicaps or defects?

Many other "danger" words that may be misleading or confusing to readers could be mentioned. Let it suffice to say that *the words we choose and the way we use them can be more important to report writing than any other single factor*. We have seen well-organized, well-planned reports that were regarded negatively by their recipients, largely because of a few inappropriate word choices.

The importance of semantic factors in clinical report writing is discussed from a legal perspective in the next chapter.

CHAPTER 8. REPORT WRITING AND THE LAW

Those who have watched television on a regular basis have become aware of a relationship that exists between the legal and medical professions. Psychiatrists and clinical psychologists are often called upon to provide testimony as to the "sanity" of a client. Medical testimony is also required in many accident cases where insurance settlements are involved. Clinicians in speech-language pathology and audiology may not have considered the possibility that they someday will have to prepare reports to be used in courts of law. They may not have thought of the possibilities of appearing in court to support the statements they have made in their reports. A number of individuals in our profession have been called upon to provide legal testimony in a variety of cases. We suspect that more of us will be called upon to do so in the future.

State licensing of speech-language pathologists and audiologists is resulting in increased involvement with legal matters, which will probably result in additional contact between members of our field and those of the legal profession.

Flower (1984, chapter 11) presents a detailed summary of legal and ethical considerations in delivering speech-language pathology and audiology services. This reference should be required reading for those preparing reports that may be used as legal testimony.

Comparatively little has been written concerning the forensic implications to the professions of speech-language pathology and audiology. Fox (1971) was one of the first to discuss the legal aspects of report writing. She states that:

> case records should be thorough and unbiased and indicate the separation of observation from opinion. The individual summoned should be prepared to substantiate his education, background and personal qualifications. Language should be easily understood and recorded in a straight-forward manner. The lawyer who has asked for the records or the witness to appear in court will usually indicate the questions he will ask during the direct examination. On cross examination the opposing attorney will question testimony or record information. There is little difficulty if the records and testimony are presented objectively. Care should be taken not to attempt to answer questions which are not within the field or to draw conclusions from insufficient data. The effort is to present evidence useful to the court in arriving at the proper decision, not to give opinion on questions for which there is no substantiating evidence (pp. 26–27)

It is of particular importance, when considering speech-language pathology and audiology reports from a legal point of view, that students and

52

professionals be knowledgeable regarding the principles of *accountability*. A publication edited by Douglass (1983), is an essential reference to provide vital information about specific applications of accountability in a variety of work settings.

Being accountable or responsible for the procedures we undertake professionally and the reporting of them accurately, is an issue that is sometimes neglected. Accountability, however, takes on great importance when speech-language pathologists are relied upon to aid in diagnosis, to predict recovery potentials, and to participate in personal injury legal cases.

Although it is always essential that we be able to justify and explain our procedures and results, our responsibility is even greater when presenting material to be dissected in the glare of legal proceedings. Speech-language pathology reports may provide important evidence contributing to decisions that pertain to monetary awards or the culpability of another party. In such cases, report writers are likely to be called upon for supportive background information regarding every evaluation instrument that has been used. It may be necessary to justify interpretations of test results and/or the conclusions of a diagnostic report.

Writing must be clear, organized, factual, and to the point. Writers should avoid cluttering reports with references to authorities, but they should be readily available when required to support conclusions at depositions or in open court.

It is wise to avoid including irrelevant data pertaining to testimony not directly related to the matter at hand. By doing so, one is likely to contribute material that can be contested or misinterpreted. It is vital that clinical reporting, presented as part of a legal proceeding, be accurate, honest, direct, thorough, and as brief and concise as possible.

A number of years ago, we were called upon by an insurance company to evaluate a 14-year-old boy who stuttered. His parents claimed that the boy's stuttering had been caused by an accident 2 years earlier, in which he had suffered a whiplash injury. After extensive medical evaluations, including psychiatric, orthopedic, and neurologic examinations, a speech-language pathology opinion was requested. The consultation report included biographical and historical information, as well as summaries of interviews with the parents and with the boy. Following a complete description of the speech mechanism examination, articulation testing, voice evaluation, language evaluation, and fluency evaluation, the report ended with the following summary and conclusions:

> The case history material available to me indicates that Robert Black had serious emotional problems prior to November 15, 1970. There is also definite evidence that he had a speech problem (lisping) prior to the accident. While there is no definite indication that stuttering symptoms were present prior to the accident, it is *not* possible to state with any degree of certainty that the accident caused the stuttering. Since emotional disturbances were present prior to November 15, 1970, Robert probably had abnormally strong emotional responses to the incident. It is possible that during this period of increased fear and tension, he may have exhibited more normal disfluencies (relaxed interruptions in the smooth

flow of speech that appear in normal speech, particularly under conditions of stress and insecurity). The parent interview revealed that his parents, and others in his environment, reacted to these repetitions and hesitations in an emotional manner, thus calling unnecessary attention to them. The stuttering behavior may have grown from Robert's attempts to inhibit these natural tension reducers. His attempts to avoid the act of stuttering have undoubtedly increased the frequency and severity of his symptoms.

The onset of stuttering usually occurs in early childhood, either during the preschool period or during the child's first years in school. The onset of stuttering in adolescence and adulthood is comparatively rare. It is possible, however, that increased awareness of symptoms already present can begin the development of a "circular response" wherein the problem grows as the individual anticipates trouble, develops apprehension and fear, becomes tense and subsequently tries to avoid exhibiting the problem to others.

I believe that if Robert's parents had been able to handle his post-accident reactions in a manner that minimized the importance of the event and if they had not responded emotionally to the normal disfluencies or beginning symptoms of stuttering at the time, he may not have become a stutterer. Had Robert been free of emotional problems at the time of the accident, he might not have responded as he did. I believe that Robert's injuries in the accident had no direct relationship to his stuttering. If there was no stuttering prior to the accident, then it must be stated that the problem developed because of emotional and social conditions which followed November 15, 1970. I believe that if the accident had not occurred, the symptoms of stuttering could have evolved from other conditions and circumstances present in his environment.

It will be noted that statements in the above report are carefully worded and that the report includes a considerable amount of information concerning the problem of stuttering, so that statements made about his parents can be more easily understood by attorneys, jury members, and the judge.

Another legal matter that has relevance to our professional written communication has to do with malpractice issues. Although malpractice suits have become increasingly more frequent among physicians and clinical psychologists, they are, fortunately, still infrequent among speech-language pathologists.

Fox (1978) discusses ways in which the risk of lawsuits can be minimized by professionals in the field of communication disorders:

> Malpractice suits against speech pathologists are rare at this time, so our guidelines come from other professions. Several suggestions for avoiding lawsuits may be appropriate. The plaintiff has the burden of proving the treatment given was not "standard." The expertise of the provider must be specified, and appropriate referral should be made if necessary skills are not present. Patients have a right to know what procedures are being suggested, and they also have the right to refuse treatment, even though this may be unwise. Always have written consent from parents or guardians before sending records to anyone, and keeping records that are adequate, up-to-date, and as complete as necessary are deterrents to possible suits. Each state has its own laws regarding "privileged communication," and knowledge of these laws may provide guidelines for what can and should be included in patient records. Above all, adequate malpractice insurance should be kept to cover these possibilities. (pp. 84–85)

Woody (1986) summarizes a variety of legal and ethical issues of concern to speech-language pathologists, particularly those in private practice.

Although not specifically concerned with report writing, Woody's chapter presents vital issues such as the practitioner-patient relationship from the point of view of legal liability. He also presents guidelines for circumventing unnecessary legal liabilities.

A text by Tallent (1988) includes a chapter entitled "Forensic Psychological Evaluations." This reference provides recommendations to psychologists who serve in court cases as expert witnesses. He states that reports to be used in forensic settings are often quite different from other types of reports. In the following statement, Tallent discusses the importance of being familiar with the legal system when preparing reports to be used in court.

> Psychologists are finding increasing acceptance in the legal forum, particularly as expert witnesses. Both research and judicial decisions support this relatively new role. To function in this forum the psychologist must acquire additional knowledge, including an understanding of the legal culture and a specialized body of legal guidelines. Psychological reports in forensic settings may in some respects differ strikingly from reports in clinics and schools, and the clinician needs special preparation to move from one area of practice to the other. A particular caution pertains to the pitfalls that are commonly encountered in psychological reporting: In the courtroom they can be a potent hazard to competent practice. (p. 222)

Tallent's chapter should be required reading for all speech-language pathologists who are considering entering the "forensic arena."

In summary, we should be certain that reports used in legal proceedings be carefully prepared, clearly written, and accurately documented. Furthermore, it is of utmost importance that professionals in the field of communication disorders be familiar with the ASHA Code of Ethics, with the principles of accountability, and with current professional literature dealing with forensic issues, to which we have referred in this chapter. In judging your own reports and progress notes it might be helpful to ask yourself the question, "Would this stand up in court?"

CHAPTER 9. ORAL REPORTING

When dealing with complex diagnostic problems and with problems that involve sensitive psychological and social implications, a written report, however well done, often seems inadequate. In such instances a telephone call and/or a conference with a physician, psychologist, teacher, another speech-language pathologist, or audiologist may be the best way to *convey* and receive information.

Klopfer (1960) points out that psychologists should not restrict their communicative efforts to formal reports. He makes this appropriate statement:

> Oral communication has many advantages as a supplement. The referent can ask questions concerning areas which have not been sufficiently clarified, he can question the psychologist as to apparent discrepancies and discover the basic unifying variables in the personality of the patient as revealed by various assessment procedures, including his own approach. In addition the personal and professional relationship between the referent and the clinical psychologist will certainly be improved by frequent contact. (pp. 2–3)

The following illustrations will suggest some of the situations in which oral supplements to written reports are needed:

1. At times we receive confidential information concerning a patient or his family. Professional ethics require that we respect the confidentiality of such personal data. We may not consider it wise to include such information in a written report. If another professional person working with this patient *needs* such data, it can be discussed more readily on the telephone or in direct communication. It is vital that a record release has been signed and that the client knows that his personal history is being discussed in confidence by two professional people who are cooperating in his treatment.

2. When a vital part of treating a patient requires that changes be made in his school environment, *direct* contact with the teacher is often necessary. Telephone conversations may be helpful, but direct contact is much more likely to attain the desired results. We routinely suggest in written reports to teachers that they call to arrange for an observation visit, so that the teacher can see and hear methods and attitudes that are involved in the treatment program of the child in question. A classroom visit by the clinician is the best way to change the attitudes of both teachers and peers toward a child with a communication problem.

It is also frequently advisable for a speech-language pathologist to communicate verbally with the principal of a school. For example, we routinely call school principals regarding classroom placement for children who stutter and for children with voice disorders. We request that the principal cooperate in the classroom placement for such children during the coming school year, selecting a teacher whose classroom tends to be relaxed and free from pressures.

Although it is not always possible to follow a written report with telephonic and/or direct conversation with the recipient of the report, it is extremely important that you *invite* such communication. This can be accomplished in the concluding paragraph of a cover letter accompanying a report or in the recommendation section of a report itself. We usually conclude such a letter to a physician or dentist by saying:

> Thank you for referring _____ to me. I will attempt to keep you informed regarding his progress. Your comments, questions and suggestions will be appreciated.
>
> Yours sincerely,

In the case of a report to teachers, we often include invitations for them to observe treatment sessions. A letter to the teacher might be concluded this way:

> I hope we will be able to work together in helping _____ with his communication problems. You are cordially invited to visit one of his treatment sessions here in the near future. Please call my office at your convenience to arrange for such a visit. I shall look forward to cooperating with you in helping _____ .
>
> Yours sincerely,

3. At times it is important to arrange a meeting of a number of professional people who are cooperating in the treatment of a person with a communicative disorder. When difficult decisions have to be made regarding a child's school placement, for example, written correspondence among the various specialists is usually inadequate. Meetings with the psychologist, physician, and school personnel, including the school speech clinician, can often be arranged.

Fisher (1969) states the importance of personal contact to public relations:

> In many cases the most effective relations are built through personal contact with individuals or groups. The clinician performs public relations whenever he discusses any aspect of his program with others. The clinician should always remember that the manner in which he works and conducts himself, and the language he uses create an impression of himself, his profession, and his program. (pp. 368–369)

In summary, if you are aware that your written report may not have accomplished all of its desired purposes, it is vital that you supplement the written report with a direct conversation with the persons for whom the report has been prepared.

CHAPTER 10. WRITING JOURNAL ARTICLES

The preceding sections of this publication may be helpful, not only in the writing of diagnostic and clinical reports, but also in the improvement of the quality of articles that are submitted to our professional journals, particularly those that deal with clinical subject matter.

The following statement by Woodford (1967) vividly summarizes the problems of contemporary scientific writing:

> In the linked worlds of experimental science, scientific editing, and science communication many scientists are considering just how serious an effect the bad writing in our journals will have on the future of science.
>
> All are agreed that the articles in our journals—even the journals with the highest standards—are, by and large, poorly written. Some of the worst are produced by the kind of author who consciously pretends to a "scientific scholarly" style. He takes what should be lively, inspiring, and beautiful, and, in an attempt to make it seem dignified, chokes it to death with stately abstract nouns; next in the name of scientific impartiality, he fits it with a complete set of passive constructions to drain away any remaining life's blood or excitement; then he embalms the remains in molasses of polysyllables, wraps the corpse in an inpenetrable vogue of words, and buries the stiff old mummy with much pomp and circumstance in the most distinguished journal that will take it. Considered either as a piece of scholarly work or as a vehicle of communication, the product is appalling. (p. 743)

The preceding statement is not offered as an example of good scientific writing but its message is so vital, it is included. Whereas it is probable that writing in the journals of the American Speech-Language-Hearing Association is generally more readable than in some scientific publications, many of our professional articles, particularly research reports, are often difficult to decipher even by those persons who are well-versed in our professional vocabulary (including jargon).

Jerger (1962) quotes a number of articles from our field that exemplify the four major problems he observes in our journal articles: Sentences are frequently too long and complicated; language is often painfully artificial; we use the passive voice to excess in verb construction; authors are discouraged from using the sparkling gems of our language, personal pronouns. (See chapter 6)

In preparing articles for publication in any of our professional journals, it is important that students and professionals pay close attention to the "information to contributors," usually located in the back of each issue. These specific requirements must be followed exactly if an article is to be considered by the editors for publication.

We suggest that after preparing a manuscript for publication you set it aside for a few days and then reread it. You will be less "involved" with the subject matter and the word patterns and probably will be more likely to discover ways of making the material more readable.

Woodford (1967) emphasizes the importance of examining one's writing at another time. He says:

> Once ideas have been written down, they can be analyzed critically and dispassionately; they can be examined at another time, in another mood, by another expert. Thoughts can therefore be developed, and if they are not precise at the first written formulation, they can be made so at a second attempt. (p. 744)

It is also advisable to have the material read by another professional person and by someone from another field who you know writes well. Such people are likely to recognize changes that should be made. After all, you know the information you want to convey, and if you find that others do not comprehend that information successfully, you must rework it before submitting it for publication.

Although this handbook is particularly aimed at report writing, many of the suggestions that have been made with respect to clinical reports apply to the preparation of journal articles. Chapter 6, "Writing Style," should be particularly applicable.

Jerger (1962) points out that our objectives in professional writing should be to inform, not to impress.

CHAPTER 11. CONCLUSIONS

This handbook has presented report-writing guidelines for students and professionals in the field of communication disorders. Our intent has been to summarize and organize pertinent information from the literature and to integrate it with our own concepts and philosophies.

We hope that the content of most sections of this handbook will be generally acceptable to professionals in the field of communication disorders. We are aware, however, that personal philosophies, theoretic points of view, and clinical attitudes vary, as they do in any profession. For example, in reviewing this handbook, we have become increasingly aware of its informality. Much of it has been written in the first person, a style with which we are comfortable, but which others may find too loose and undignified. Certainly, excellent reports have been written in the third person. We hope that those who teach their students a more formal writing style or a different organizational format, will still find *Report Writing* to be a helpful reference. Our years in private practice have taught us many valuable lessons pertaining to the ethical, semantic, and legal aspects of report writing. We have attempted to share them with you, the reader, as simply and concisely as possible.

In his text, *Psychological Report Writing*, Tallent (1988) provides a "Quality Check of the Psychological Report." This checklist is made up of the following list of questions which are directly applicable to the field of speech-language pathology:

Does the report meet all responsibilities, ethical and legal, to the client, and to the community, and, as applicable, to other professionals and agencies?

Is the completion of the report timely?

Is the report properly focused in terms of the reason for assessment, data on the client, and a frame of reference?

Does the content unnecessarily duplicate that of others? (Is there encroachment on the establishment role of other professions?)

If raw data are presented, is the material also interpreted or used for illustration?

Is all appropriate illustrative material presented?

Is all of the content relevant and significant?

Is content presented with appropriate emphasis?

Are diagnoses, prognoses, and recommendations given as necessary?

Is all other essential material included?

Is interpretation sufficiently focused (not too general, differentiating among clients)?

Are conclusions adequately supported by data?

Is speculation within reason?

Is speculation properly labeled as such?

Are all interpretations within acceptable levels of responsibility?

Is the report written so as to be meaningful and useful?

Are exhibitionistic, authoritative, or similarly offensive statements avoided?

Is the report client-oriented rather than test-oriented?

Are concepts that are too theoretical or too abstract avoided?

Is word usage appropriate (absence or jargon, stereotyped, esoteric, overly technical, or complex language)?

Is the language used clear and unambiguous?

Is the report too long (padded, redundant, rambling, unfocused, offering useless content, or in the manner of a "shotgun approach")?

Is the style appropriate for the mission, for the setting, and for those who may read it?

Is the report logically and effectively organized?

Are the conclusions of the report set forth without hedging?

Is the report adequately persuasive in terms of needs and forcefulness of the data?

Is the report self-contradictory? (p. 244)

If we can answer "yes" to most of these questions, we are well on our way to success as report writers.

In reading the varied sources that have been included in the bibliography, many of which we have used as references in the text, we have broadened our own concepts of report writing. We encourage both students and professionals to make use of information included in this handbook as well as information contained in the references listed in the bibliography. If this handbook improves the readability of the reports that represent our profession, our purpose will have been accomplished.

REFERENCES

AMERICAN SPEECH-LANGUAGE-HEARING ASSOCIATION (1983). Professional Services Board: Standards for PSB accreditation. *Asha, 25,* 51–58.

AMERICAN SPEECH-LANGUAGE-HEARING ASSOCIATION (1983). Professional Services Board: Organization and Maintenance of records for clinical and service delivery. *Asha 26*(4), 49.

AMERICAN SPEECH AND HEARING ASSOCIATION, (1975). PSROs: A manual for speech pathologists and audiologists.

AVERILL, R. W. (1974). Implications of PSRO to independent health professions. *Asha, 16,* 677–679.

BANGS, T. (1961). Evaluating children with language delay. *Journal of Speech and Hearing Disorders, 36,* 6–18.

BANGS, T., & RISTER, A. (1969). Efficiency in report writing. *Hearing and Speech News, 37,* 12–16.

BARRIE-BLACKLEY, S., MUSSELWHITE, C. R., & ROGISTER, S. H. (1978). *Clinical oral language sampling.* Danville, IL: Interstate.

BEARDSLEY, M. C. (1966). *Thinking straight* (3rd edition). Englewood Cliffs, NJ: Prentice-Hall.

BILLINGS, B. L., & SCHMITZ, H. D. (1980). *Report writing in audiology.* Danville, IL: Interstate.

BLACK, M. E. (1964). *Speech correction in the schools.* Englewood Cliffs, NJ: Prentice-Hall.

BLUHM, M. (1987). *The doctor goes to court.* (3rd edition). Rancho Mirage, CA: Michael Bluhm, Publisher.

BUTLER, K. G. (Ed.). (1986). *Prospering in private practice.* Rockville, MD: Aspen.

CHAPMAN, M. E. (1969). The speech clinician - as a professional person. In R. J. Van Hattum (Ed.), *Clinical speech in the schools.* Springfield, IL: Charles C. Thomas.

CHIAL, M. R. (1984). Glossary of microcomputer terms. In A. H. Schwartz (Ed.) (chapter 13). *Handbook of microcomputer applications in communication disorders.* San Diego, CA: College-Hill Press.

Code of Ethics of the American Speech-Language-Hearing Association (1987). (revised January 1, 1986). *Asha, 29* (3), 59–61.

DARLEY, F. L. (1964). *Diagnosis and appraisal of communication disorders.* Englewood Cliffs, NJ: Prentice-Hall.

DAWSON W. L. (1973). *Instrumentation in the speech clinic, A handbook for clinicians and students.* Danville, IL: Interstate.

DOUGLASS, R. L. (Ed.). (1983). Clinical accountability: Schools, clinics, private practice. *Seminars in speech and language, 4* (2), 107–184.

DOWNEY, M., WHITE, S., & KARR, S. (1984). *Health insurance manual for speech-language pathologists and audiologists.* Rockville, MD: American Speech-Language-Hearing Association.

DUBLINSKE, S. (1978). PL 94-142: Developing the individualized education program (IEP). *Asha, 20,* 380–397.

EHRLICH, E., & MURPHY, D. (1964). *The art of technical writing.* New York: Thomas Y. Crowell Co.

ELBOW, P. (1981). *Writing with power.* New York: Oxford.

EMERICK, L. (1969). *The parent interview, Guidelines for students and practicing speech clinicians.* Danville, IL: Interstate.

EMERICK, L. L., & HAYNES, W. O. (1986). *Diagnosis and evaluation in speech pathology* (3rd edition). Englewood Cliffs, NJ: Prentice-Hall.

ENGLISH H. B., & ENGLISH A. C. (1958). *A comprehensive dictionary of psychological and psychoanalytical terms.* New York: Longmars, Green.

ENGLISH, R. E., & LILLYWHITE, H. S. (1963). A semantic approach to clinical reporting in speech pathology. *Asha, 5,* 647–650.

EWING, D. W., (1974). *Writing for results in business, government, the sciences, and the professions* (2nd edition). New York: John Wiley & Sons.

FISHER, L. I. (1969). Reporting: In the schools to the community. In R. J. Van Hattum (Ed.), *Clinical speech in the schools.* Springfield, IL: Charles C. Thomas.

FITCH, J. L., DAVIS, L. A., EVANS, W. B., & SELLERS, D. E. (1984). Computer-managed screening for communication disorders. *Language, Speech, and Hearing Services in Schools, 15,* 66–69.

FLOWER, R. (Ed.). (1984). *Delivery of speech-language pathology and audiology services.* Baltimore: Williams & Wilkins.

FLOWER, R. (1985). Asking questions (presidential address). *Asha, 27* (12), 21–23.

FOWLER, H. W. (1986). *Modern English usage* (2nd edition). New York: Oxford University Press.

FOX, D. R. (Ed.). (1971). *Private practice, guidelines for speech pathology and audiology.* Danville, IL: Interstate.

FOX, D. R. (1978). Forensic speech pathology. In R. R. Battin & D. R. Fox, *Private practice in audiology and speech pathology.* New York: Grune & Stratton.

GOOD, R. (1970). The written language of rehabilitation medicine: Meaning and usages. *Archives of Physical Medicine and Rehabilitation, 15,* 29–36.

GOWER, E. (1954). *Plain words.* New York: Knopf.

GRAVES, H. F., & HOFFMAN, L. S. S. (1965). *Report writing* (4th edition). Englewood Cliffs, NJ: Prentice-Hall.

HAMMOND, K. R., & ALLEN, J. M., JR. (1953). *Writing clinical reports.* New York: Prentice-Hall.

HAYNES, W. C., & HARTMAN, D. E. (1975). The agony of report writing: a new look at an old problem. *Journal of the National Student Speech and Hearing Association, 3,* (1), 7–15.

HOOD, S. B., & MILLER, L. R. (1984). Administrative applications for microcomputers (Chapter 10). In A. H. Schwartz (Ed.), *Handbook of microcomputer applications in communication disorders*. San Diego, CA: College-Hill Press.

HOULE, G. R. (1988). Computer usage by speech-language pathologists in public schools. *Language, Speech, and Hearing Services in Schools, 19*, (4), 423–427.

HUBER, J. T. (1969). *Report writing in psychology and psychiatry*. New York: Harper & Row.

HYMAN, C. (1986). The 1985 omnibus survey. *Asha, 28* (4), 19–22.

HYMAN C. (1987). The 1986–1987 omnibus survey. *Asha, 29* (8), 29–33.

IRWIN, R. B. (1969). *Speech and hearing therapy*. Pittsburgh: Stanwix House.

JERGER, J. (1962). Scientific writing can be reasonable. *Asha, 4*, 191–204.

JOHNSON, W. (1946). *People in quandaries*. New York: Harper & Row.

JOHNSON, W., DARLEY, F. L. & SPRIESTERSBACH, D. (1961). *Diagnostic methods in speech pathology*. New York: Harper & Bros.

JOHNSON, W. P. (1971). *Writing scientific papers and reports* (6th ed.). Dubuque, IA: Wm. C. Brown.

KAMARA, C. (1986). ASHA's professional practice activities. *Asha, 28* (9), 25–27.

KING, R. R., & BERGER, K. W. (1971). *Diagnostic assessment and counseling techniques for speech pathologists and audiologists*. Pittsburgh: Stanwix House.

KLOPFER, W. G. (1960). *The psychological report*. New York: Grune & Stratton.

KNEPFLAR, K. J. (1972). Is full-time private practice for you? *California Journal of Communicative Disorders, 2*, 143–146.

KNEPFLAR, K. J. (1978). Report writing for private practitioners. In R. Battin & D. Fox. (Eds.), *Private practice in audiology and speech pathology*. New York: Grune & Stratton.

KNEPFLAR, K. J. (1973/October). *The private practitioner's accountability under ASHA's code of ethics*. Unpublished paper presented at ASHA Convention, Detroit, MI.

KRUEGER, B. (1985). Computerized reporting in a public school program. *Language, Speech, and Hearing in Schools, 16* (2), 135–139.

LAGUAITE, J., RIVIERE, M., & FULLER, C. (1965). Problems of terminology. *Asha, 7*, 152–155.

LEHRHOFF, I., & KOROSHEC, S. (1980). *Speech and language procedure manual*. Beverly Hills, CA: Irwin Lehrhoff.

MACK, K., & SKJEI, E. (1979). *Overcoming writing blocks*. Los Angeles, CA: J. P. Tarcher.

MAYMAN, M. (1959). Style, focus language and content of an ideal psychologic test report. *Journal of projective techniques, 23*, 453.

MERRILL, P. W. (1947). The principles of poor writing. *Scientific Monthly, 64*, 72-74.

MILLER, T. B., & LUBINSKI, R. (1986). Professional liability in speech-language pathology and audiology. *Asha, 28* (6), 45–47.

MOORE, M. V. (1969). Pathological writing. *Asha, 11,* 535–538.

MORRIS, W., & MORRIS, M. (1975). *Harper dictionary of contemporary usage.* New York: Harper & Row.

MURPHY, A. T. (1974). The quiet hyena: Two monologues in search of a dialogue. In L. L. Emerick & S. B. Hood, (Ed.), *The client-clinician relationship* (Chapter 2). Springfield, IL: Thomas.

NATION, J. E., & ARAM, D. M. (1977). *Diagnosis of speech and language disorders.* St. Louis: C. V. Mosby.

NEWTON, M. (1986). Computer applications in private practice: Getting started. In K. G. Butler (Ed.), *Prospering in private practice.* (Chapter 10). Rockville, MD: Aspen.

NEWTON, M. (1986). Standard computer software applications in private practice, Chapter 13 in K. G. Butler (Ed.), *Prospering in private practice* (Chapter 13). Rockville, MD: Aspen.

NICOLOSI, L., HARRYMAN E., & KRESHECK, J. (1983). *Terminology in communication disorders: Speech-language-hearing.* Baltimore: William & Wilkins.

PANNBACKER, M. (1975). Diagnostic report writing. *Journal of Speech and Hearing Disorders, 40,* 367–379.

PROFESSIONAL LIABILITY INSURANCE (1966). Announcement. *Asha, 8,* 47.

RILEY, G. D. (1981). *Stuttering Prediction Instrument for Young Children.* Austin, TX: Pro-Ed, Inc.

RILEY, G. D. (1980). *Stuttering Severity Instrument for Children and Adults.* Austin, TX: Pro-Ed, Inc.

RUSHAKOFF, G. E. (1984). Clinical applications in communication disorders. In A. H. Schwartz (Ed.), *Handbook of microcomputer applications in communication disorders* (Chapter 1). San Diego, CA: College-Hill Press.

RUSHAKOFF, G. E., & LOMBARDINO, L. J. (1984). Microcomputer applications. *Asha, 26* (6), 27–31.

SANDERS, L. (1972). *Evaluation of speech and language disorders in children.* Danville, IL: Interstate.

SCHWARTZ, A. H. (Ed.). (1984). *Handbook of microcomputer applications in communication disorders.* San Diego, CA: College-Hill Press.

SHAW, H. (1975). *Dictionary of problem words and expression.* New York: McGraw-Hill.

SHERTZER, M. (1986). *The elements of grammar.* New York: Macmillan.

SIEGEL, G. M. (1975). The high cost of accountability. *Asha, 17,* 796–797.

SISSON, A. F. (1975). *Sisson's word and expression locater.* West Nyack, NY: Parker Publishing.

SKILLEN, M. E., & GAY, R. M. (1974). *Words into type* (3rd edition). Englewood Cliffs, NJ: Prentice-Hall.

STEVENS, N. E. (1950). The moral obligation to be intelligible. *Scientific Monthly, 70,* 111–115.

STRUNK, W., JR., & WHITE, E. B. (1979). *The elements of style* (3rd edition). New York: MacMillan.

TALLENT, N. (1958). On individualizing the psychologist's clinical evaluation. *Journal of Clinical Psychology, 14,* 243–245.

TALLENT, N. (1988). *Psychological report writing* (3rd edition). Englewood Cliffs, NJ: Prentice-Hall.

THOMPSON, E. T. (Ed.). (1961). *Standard nomenclature of diseases and operations* (5th edition). New York: McGraw-Hill.

VAN HAGEN, C. E. (1961). *Report writers handbook.* Englewood Cliffs, NJ: Prentice-Hall.

VAN RIPER, C., & DOPHEIDE, W. (1966). Diagnostic services in a training center. *Asha, 8,* 37–39.

WEISS, C. E., GORDON, M. E., & LILLYWHITE, H. S. (1987). *Clinical management of articulatory and phonologic disorders* (2nd edition). Baltimore: Williams & Wilkins.

WILBUR, L. A. (1977). Use of the problem oriented medical record in the speech and hearing profession. *Asha, 19* (3), 157–159.

WOLFE, D. (1967). Bad writing. *Science, 155,* 407.

WOODFORD, F. P. (1967). Sounder thinking through clear writing. *Science, 156,* 743–744.

WOODY, R. H. (1986). Legal issues for private practicioners in speech-language pathology and audiology. In K. G. Butler, (Ed.), *Prospering in private practice.* Rockville, MD: Aspen.

WRIGHT, R. H. (1981). What to do until the malpractice lawyer comes: A survivor's manual. *American Psychologist, 36* (12), 1535–1541.

APPENDIX A

LETTERS AND SUGGESTIONS TO TEACHERS

Example of letter to elementary schoolteacher of a child who stutters

September 19, 1985

Mrs. J. C. Wright
Fourth Grade Teacher
Pasadena Elementary School
Pasadena, California

Dear Mrs. Wright:

I am currently seeing Jack Strong for treatment of his stuttering problem. Stuttering is a frequently misunderstood disorder, with causes and symptoms varying from patient to patient. As part of my work with stutterers, I attempt to cooperate closely with teachers.

A few of the basic points that should be considered by teachers of young people who stutter are included on the enclosed list of suggestions. Frequently without realizing it, teachers are reinforcing stutterers' attempts to cover up stuttering and to avoid speaking situations. Jack's treatment involves facing speaking situations and learning to deal with the problem rather than avoiding it.

Mr. and Mrs. Strong are cooperating closely with our treatment program. I welcome you to our team. In some instances I arrange for classroom visits to assist stutterers in overcoming fears and to assist teachers and classmates in understanding the problem. I would be happy to speak to you personally about Jack. If you have comments or questions, please feel free to call.

Yours sincerely,

Clinician's name and degree
Speech-Language Pathologist

Suggestions to classroom teachers of children who stutter

Kenneth J. Knepflar, Ph.D.
Private Practice
Pasadena, California

Many teachers have unintentionally increased the problems of those who stutter, often with all good intentions of helping. The following suggestions are applicable not only for stutterers, but for other shy, sensitive, or fearful children who may be present in any classroom, often sitting quietly in a corner without anyone knowing the feelings of inadequacy they are experiencing.

1. Expect stutterers to fulfill all speaking responsibilities in the classroom. Not calling on them or allowing them to do written work instead of speaking increases their feelings of being different.
2. Keep "eye contact" with stutterers and encourage them to look at the person to whom they are speaking. This assures them of your interest and encourages them to face their problem.
3. Do not fill in words when stutterers are "stuck." By doing so, you provide a crutch and increase their feelings that they cannot talk for themselves.
4. Do not pretend that you do not notice an obvious problem. If you do, students are likely to think that the problem is too shameful to be discussed or that you are too embarrassed to mention it. Talk openly about stuttering, just as you would any other problem that children have. A broken arm, a recent disease, a reading difficulty are talkable; so should stuttering be. Explain that stutterers try hard to speak too perfectly and that we all repeat sounds, words, and phrases at times. Stress the importance of facing any problem that we may have.
5. Help those who tease and mimic stutterers to understand that they are not perfect either and they are pointing out someone else's problem instead of facing their own.
6. Do not place children who stutter under unnecessary time pressure. If a child is working or talking as rapidly as he can, his problem will be complicated when he feels rushed.
7. Do not call on students in alphabetical order or in the order they are seated in the classroom. Stutterers anticipate that they will stutter and the longer they wait as their turn approaches, the more tension they are likely to build.
8. Call on stutterers early in a class period so that they will not have time to build unnecessary fears and tension.
9. Do not praise periods of spontaneous fluency. Often stutterers do not know why they have a "good day" when their speech happens to be normal. By praising the fluency you increase the stutterer's desire to maintain a steady flow of words. Then the next time he stutters, he holds back even more trying to please you, thus building additional tension.
10. Try to be interested in *what* each child has to say. If a person who

stutters knows you respect his intelligence, his ideas, and his attitudes, his self-concept is greatly improved, and he is more likely to approach speaking situations.

11. If a stutterer is a poor reader, asking him to read aloud can be a highly feared situation for him. Help with reading, then, is the only way oral reading can become more fluent. Some stutterers experience their first real speaking tension during early oral reading situations. When reading is introduced before a child has acquired the necessary readiness skills, feelings of failure and frustration inevitably result.

12. Be aware of your own speech. If you speak too rapidly or with language structure and vocabulary that is above the child's level of comprehension, you are building tension and setting unrealistic goals for the child.

13. Attempt to maintain an objective attitude concerning all of your students and their problems. This is particularly important with respect to stutterers. *Students need your understanding, not your sympathy or pity.*

14. The struggle for an unrealistic level of speaking fluency is often not the only perfectionistic or compulsive aspect of the behavior of those who stutter. Try not to build unnecessary tension and frustration by insisting upon levels of perfection in handwriting, art, or athletic activities that are beyond the student's capacity.

Example of letter to teacher of a child with vocal nodules

Mrs. Mary Clark
Franklin Elementary School
Los Angeles, California

Dear Mrs. Clark:

As you may know, Bob James, who currently attends your third-grade class, is under treatment for a voice disorder. Bob has been seen by John Johnson, M.D. who has diagnosed that Bob has vocal nodules, which are small fibrous growths on the surfaces of the vocal cords. They are caused by habitual misuse and strain of the voice. This kind of voice problem in children should be treated by vocal rest and voice training by a qualified speech-language pathologist. When nodules are not treated, they often become worse and then require surgery. Even when surgery is done, vocal rehabilitation services are usually necessary to prevent their return.

The aims of Bob's treatment program are to raise his habitual pitch level slightly, teach him an easier, more natural way of initiating voice, altering his breathing habits for speaking and reducing his speaking rate.

Until Bob has completed his vocal training, it is extremely important that you be aware of his voice in the classroom. He should be discouraged from loud screaming and shouting on the playground. For the time being, he should not participate in classroom singing activities.

In addition to his voice disorder, Bob exhibits other evidences of tension. His art work, for example, shows overly precise, compulsively neat behavior with very little freedom of movement. He needs to learn to accept more freedom and less perfection in many of his activities. It is particularly important for Bob to be in a classroom environment that is free from unnecessary tension and pressure.

I hope you will be able to cooperate with Bob's vocal rehabilitation program. Your comments and questions will be appreciated.

Yours sincerely,

Clinician's name and degree,
Speech-Language Pathologist

Example of a letter to teacher of a college student who stutters

October 17, 1987

Mr. John Thomas, Instructor
Los Angeles City College
Vermont Street
Los Angeles, California

Dear Mr. Thomas:

My patient, Mr. Joe Green, is a student in one of your classes. Joe has been receiving speech therapy under my direction since March, 1986. In order for treatment to be of maximum benefit to stutterers, it is frequently necessary for me to communicate with teachers so that clinical progress can be carried over efficiently into outside speaking situations. I welcome this opportunity to discuss with you some of the details of Joe's problem and his treatment program.

At the time of his initial evaluation, Joe's stuttering symptoms were extremely severe. Most of his attempts to speak resulted in struggle reactions including eye closures, facial grimaces, tongue clicks, head jerks, and extreme breath holding. Joe has stuttered since early childhood, but the problem increased in severity during high school and his first year of college.

His problem developed partially because of his attempts to please his listeners and to speak more fluently than his capacity would allow. His "tricks" to try to avoid stuttering became habituated and added to the complexity of his symptoms.

Joe has made outstanding progress in treatment. He now faces speaking situations that were formerly avoided. In most situations he is able to speak with less frequent moments of stuttering and with much less severe struggle behavior. In other words, he has learned to handle the problem rather than to run away from it. He has also learned to accept the fact that normal speech is not perfectly fluent (that it contains interjections of uh, well, er, you know, etc., as well as word and phrase repetitions).

His most severe stuttering continues to be present under circumstances in which he feels his listeners do not accept his stuttering and when he responds unfavorably to time pressures. He frequently experiences these kinds of difficulties in classroom situations.

I communicated frequently last year with Joe's instructions at the college, which resulted in his presenting speeches on stuttering to a number of psychology and public speaking classes. Such experiences decreased his fears of speaking situations and increased his confidence in himself as a communicator.

Enclosed is a list of suggestions to teachers of stutterers, which you may find of interest. I sincerely hope that this letter will assist you in understanding Joe's communicative problem. I believe he is a bright, highly motivated young man and I am optimistic concerning his prognosis for continued improvement.

Thank you for your cooperation.

Yours sincerely,

Clinician's name and degree
Title

APPENDIX B

RECORDS RELEASE FORMS
EVALUATION REPORTS
SPECIALIZED CASE HISTORY FORMS
DIAGNOSTIC REPORT LETTER
CONSULTATION REPORT
TEST PROTOCOL
DIAGNOSTIC CODES
COMPUTERIZED DIAGNOSTIC SUMMARY

RECORDS RELEASE

Date _____

To _____

_____

I hereby authorize you to release to

_____

_____

any information including the diagnosis and records of any treatment or examination rendered to me during the period from _____ to _____

_____
SIGNATURE

_____
WITNESS

NO. 3341 COLWELL CO., CHAMPAIGN, ILL.

73

REQUEST FOR AND CONSENT TO RELEASE OF INFORMATION
FROM PATIENT'S RECORDS

NOTE.— The execution of this form does not authorize the release of information other than that specifically enumerated herein.

TO

NAME

SOCIAL SECURITY NUMBER

I here request and authorize to release the following information, from the records identified above to:

INFORMATION REQUESTED (Number each item requested and give the dates or approximate dates—period from and to—covered by each.)

PURPOSES FOR WHICH THE INFORMATION IS TO BE USED

NOTE.— Additional items of information desired may be listed on the reverse hereof.

DATE

SIGNATURE AND ADDRESS OF PATIENT OR GUARDIAN

Example of an evaluation report for a patient with Parkinson's Disease

EVALUATION REPORT

Name: Charles Smith   Birthdate: March 21, 1920   Age: 55
Address: 5984 E. First Street, Los Angeles, California
Evaluation date: September 20, 1975
Referred by: John Jones, M.D.

Reason for Referral: Patient has become unintelligible, even to his wife. Evaluation was requested to establish prognosis for improving intelligibility.

Background Information: According to information provided by Mr. Smith and his wife, who accompanied him to the evaluation, the patient's Parkinson's Disease was first diagnosed almost twenty five years ago. His first symptoms were hand tremors and head shaking. Mr. Smith has undergone three surgical procedures. The first surgery (about twelve years ago) stopped much of the tremors and had no significant adverse effects. The second surgery (two years later) also had good results. The third procedure (one year after the second) resulted in some complications including impaired speech and decreased leg function.

Mr. Smith, an attorney, continued working until about five years ago, when he retired, largely because of his speech impairment. Mr. Smith stated that while his speech has been reasonably stable during the past six years, he believes he has probably become gradually less intelligible during that period of time.

Hearing Evaluation: Pure-tone audiometric testing revealed that Mr. Smith's auditory acuity is within normal limits.

Speech Mechanism: Mr. Smith's oral structures are essentially within normal limits. All lip, tongue, velar, and mandibular functions are possible, but noticeably more labored and less accurate than normal. The repetitive rate of movement of the lips, tongue, and mandible is significantly below normal limits. Velar action is sluggish.

Articulation: On an isolated word articulation test, Mr. Smith can produce most of the consonant and vowel sounds within normal limits. Inconsistent moderate distortions of the s, z, sh, ch, j and the th sounds were observed. This suggests impaired fine muscle tongue function, resulting in inadequate control of the air stream during attempts to produce these sounds.

A significant degree of breakdown occurs on many of the consonant sounds during attempts at conversational speech. The consonant blends, particularly the sk, skw, st, str, sl, and spl are frequently inaccurate.

Voice: Mr. Smith's habitual speaking voice is usually inaudible. His loudness is limited; his speaking pitch, abnormally high; and his quality moderately breathy and hoarse. His maximum phonation time of 26 seconds indicates a better ability for controlling the air stream over the vocal folds than his habitual speaking patterns indicate. His voice problem interferes with communication more than his articulation.

Language: There are no evidences of organic language disabilities in this patient at this time.

Rate and Fluency: At times, Mr. Smith is slightly disfluent, probably more because of frustration and his awareness of his communication failures than because of any of the organic factors that are present. His habitual speaking rate is too rapid for his current level of neuromuscular functioning. It is probable that he is attempting to maintain his old speaking rate. Mr. Smith's speaking attempts are much more intelligible and audible when he slows his rate.

Psychological Factors: While it is obvious that Mr. Smith is frustrated and somewhat depressed at times, he has maintained much of his sense of humor and emotional strength.

Clinical Impressions: Mr. Smith has a severe voice disorder and a moderately severe articulation problem caused by Parkinson's Disease. While normal communicative skills are undoubtedly out of the question for this patient, I believe that his articulation and voice functioning can be helped by means of a planned home exercise program, and a limited treatment program emphasizing rate control and improved control of the respiratory musculature.

Recommendations: Mr. Smith has been scheduled for one, one-half hour treatment session weekly. I anticipate reducing the frequency of his visits to once monthly after six weeks, when a home treatment program should be functioning well for him.

Clinician's name and degree,
Speech Pathologist

Example of evaluation report of a child who stutters

Name: Douglas Frank
Birthdate: August 23, 1964   Age: 10 years, 10 months
Date of Evaluation: June 25, 1975

Background Information: Douglas began speaking a few words at the age of 11 months, but he had very little speech during the first two years of life. His early speech and language development was apparently within normal limits, although his mother stated that he substituted (y) for the (l) sound. She said that she "bribed" him to correct the sound. Doug's parents agreed that stuttering symptoms first appeared at the age of 4 during his last year of preschool. At that time, their pediatrician recommended that they "let it ride," which they did.

Mr. and Mrs. Frank do not believe that they have called attention to Doug's stuttering. They have not said "slow down," "think before you talk," "take a deep breath" or any of the kinds of corrective labeling statements that so often occur in the speech environments of young stutterers. It is important to note, however, that Mr. Frank also stutters. While his symptoms are severe, he totally avoided discussing the subject during the interview.

Douglas has not received treatment for his stuttering in elementary school. Doug and his family received a limited amount of counseling in the office of John Jackson, Ph.D., a speech pathologist in Los Angeles. This treatment was discontinued by the parents who believed it was not meeting Doug's needs.

According to his parents, Douglas has had understanding teachers who have handled him well. As far as they know, he has not been teased because of his stuttering.

Hearing: Pure tone air and bone audiometric testing revealed that Doug's auditory acuity is normal.

Speech Mechanism: With the exception of a mild orthodontic problem, Doug's speech mechanism is completely within normal limits.

Articulation: No formal articulation test was administered. Doug's articulation of speech sounds is completely within normal limits, however, as revealed by an informal evaluation during the interview.

Language: On Form A of the Peabody Picture Vocabulary Test, Douglas scored at the 16 year, 7 month level, which at a chronological age of 10 years, 10 months indicates highly superior vocabulary comprehension. He was prone to guess throughout the test, which suggests that his actual vocabulary of recognition may be slightly below his performance on this test. Nevertheless, it is apparent that his comprehension of language is superior.

Doug's conversational speech revealed no evidence of expressive language problems. His vocabulary, sentence structure, grammar, and syntax appear to be in the upper limits of the normal range.

Voice: Doug's voice, at this time, is within normal limits acoustically, except during moments of stuttering, which are characterized by laryngeal struggle and noticeable disruptions in respiratory function. Moments of stuttering are frequently accompanied by brief upper thoracic inhalations.

Fluency: Doug's speaking fluency is significantly impaired both in conversational speech and oral reading. His secondary stuttering symptoms include eye blinks, tense single phoneme repetitions, tense silent pauses preceding stuttered words, and rapidly spoken interjections of phrases such as "hold it" and "you know" which serve as starters preceding moments of stuttering.

Doug's periods of "normal speech" are usually fluent with little evidence of normal disfluency.

Clinical Impressions: Douglas exhibits moderately severe secondary stuttering symptoms. His avoidances of stuttering are largely at the word level, however, with few complete avoidances of actual speaking situations. His outgoing personality has apparently been preserved thus far, in spite of the stuttering.

Doug's high vocabulary score indicates that he is probably aspiring for a high level of verbal functioning, which is being frustrated by his stuttering. He appears to be highly sensitive and very impatient with himself. It appears that the subject of stuttering has been a rather closed topic in the Frank household. (Douglas seemed relieved to be able to talk openly about his stuttering during our interview.)

Recommendations:

1. Douglas should be seen during the next school year by a competent speech pathologist.
2. It would be of great benefit to Douglas if his father also were to receive treatment for his stuttering.
3. A continuing program of parent counseling should be planned for Mr. and Mrs. Frank.

Example of a brief evaluation report of a laryngectomized patient (suitable to submit with an insurance claim)

SPEECH EVALUTION REPORT

NAME: Hart, Arthur   AGE: 61
DATE OF INITIAL EVALUATION: 6/1/87
REFERRED BY: Roger Roy, M.D., California Medical Center
DIAGNOSIS: Total aphonia (absence of voice) following total laryngec-
tomy and left radical neck dissection on May 19, 1987.

Background Information: Mr. Hart first experienced symptoms of hoarseness in November, 1986. After several other medical consultations, the patient was seen at California Medical Center by Dr. Roger Roy, who diagnosed carcinoma of the right lung, as well as cancer of the larynx. In April, 1987, a right upper lobectomy was performed by a thoracic surgeon at U.C.L.A. and on May 19, 1987, he underwent a total laryngectomy and a left radical neck dissection. Mr. Hart was seen for his initial speech consultation less than two weeks following his laryngectomy. Postsurgical radiation is to be conducted during the next six weeks.

Evaluation Findings: Mr. Hart is totally without voice as the result of his surgery. During his first session several electrolarynx devices were demonstrated. He used the Cooper Rand electrolarynx easily because it did not interfere with postsurgical neck tenderness. This device was loaned to him until he selects another device and until successful esophageal speech training is accomplished.

Mr. Hart responded positively to initial tests using the plosive sounds p, t, and k. He was able to inject air into the upper esophagus and produced a quiet, pleasant sounding esophageal voice on p, t, and k syllables. He successfully inhibited stoma noise during his initial practice session.

Prognosis: On the basis of Mr. Hart's response to his evaluation session, his prognosis for developing efficient esophageal speech is excellent.

Recommendations: Mr. Hart should be seen for two individual esophageal voice therapy sessions weekly to start. The frequency of his sessions will be reduced as progress allows.

Clinician's name and degree,
Title(s)

Example of a report of a thorough evaluation of language/learning skills of an 8-year-old

LEARNING ABILITY EVALUATION

NAME: Dean Rodney
BIRTH DATE: 04/20/78
TEST DATE: 02/20/87
C. A.: 8-10

Referral and Background: Dean was referred by Walter Kennedy, M.D., his Pediatrician. Dean is an eight-year-old, right-handed male, in a special education program in school. Dr. Kennedy reports that Dean has a history of dyslexia and hyperactive behavior. Diagnosis and prognosis were requested, regarding factors contributing to the dyslexia and problems of attention, concentration, and academic performance.

Tests Administered

Peabody Picture Vocabulary Test	8-7	Mental Age
Woodcock Reading Mastery Test		
Word Attack	Unable to Score	
Slosson Oral Reading Test	.7	Grade Level
Wide Range Achievement Test		
Reading	1B	Grade Level
Spelling	1B	Grade Level
Arithmetic	2B	Grade Level
Gray Oral Reading Test	Unable to Score	
Detroit Tests of Learning Aptitude		
Verbal Absurdities	11-0	Mental Age
Verbal Opposites	10-0	Mental Age
Designs	7-6	Mental Age
Auditory Attention for Related Syllables	6-9	Mental Age
Visual Memory for Letters	7-6	Mental Age
Oral Directions	7-9	Mental Age
Lindamood Auditory Conceptualization Test	40/100	
Informal Tests of Writing		
Sound/Symbol Associations	19/32	
Syllable Contrasts	0/3	

Summary and Conclusions: Dean was distractible in the testing situation, but undertook each task as it was presented and with encouragement, appeared to go to the limit of his ability. A central nervous system dysfunction in auditory conceptualization was identified that has significantly interfered with Dean's processing of written language. The dysfunction is preventing this intelligent boy from grasping the relationship between oral and written language, and is making it virtually impossible for him to acquire written language skills which are commensurate with his oral language skills. He is appropriately classified under ICD-9 781.9, with symptoms involving nervous and muscular-skeletal systems processing dysfunction.

The auditory conceptual dysfunction that has been identified responds to specific treatment procedures, and the prognosis is good for successful treatment of both the primary sensory dysfunction and the sensory disabilities in reading and spelling resulting from it.

Specific Functions: Auditory memory for sentences is two years below age-expectancy. Visual memory for letters is more than one year below. However, when the two modalities are combined, visual input supports auditory input for Dean, enabling him to perform at the lower end of the normal range in Oral Directions.

In auditory conceptual function, Dean correctly conceptualized the identity, number, and sequence of isolated sounds spoken in a pattern, but he demonstrates severe difficulty in making these same judgments about sounds spoken in syllables. When syllables of two or more sounds are changed by the addition, omission, substitution, or shift of one sound, he is unable to accurately perceive the nature of these changes. The adverse effect of this primary sensory disorder on Dean's reading and spelling, and also on his semantic associations, will be indicated below. It is a very important factor in the written language problems he is experiencing.

Oral Language: Dean's receptive vocabulary is at an average level, but his auditory conceptual disorder causes semantic confusions. Dean confuses words that are closely similar in sound structure (e.g., mound and mount). Obviously, word confusions such as these can also adversely affect language comprehension at a given moment.

In a measure of verbal absurdities, Dean's total score is above age-expectancy, but his performance was spotty, and successes and failures were spread over a considerable range. He required repetitions of several anecdotes before he could respond. Dean is also presently limited in his ability to engage in further vocabulary building activity through reading, as would normally occur.

Written Language: Dean's reading skills center around the first-grade level, depending on the tasks involved. His performance within this range is marked repeatedly by the influence of his auditory disorder. Because he is unable to monitor the sound-letter incompatibilities involved, he is unable to perceive and self-correct such errors as "house" for *here*, "beetle" for *deep*, "balls" for *spell*, etc. This is also the case with spelling "hab" for *and*, "caume" for *cook*, "lut" for *light*, etc.

In two measures of reading comprehension, Dean performed significantly below the level of his oral vocabulary. There was evidence that the inaccurate decoding discussed above was a factor in Dean's comprehension problems.

His auditory dysfunction makes it extremely difficult for him to monitor and successfully attack unfamiliar words when they occur in his reading, causing him to skip over them.

Impression and Prognosis: Dean has a severe central nervous system dysfunction in processing the phonological aspect of language, which in turn contributes to secondary problems with the morphological, syntactic, and semantic aspects of spoken and written language. The prognosis is good for significant improvement in all four areas of processing if the recommendations for treatment are followed.

Recommendations:
1. Treatment for auditory conceptual dysfunction should be initiated immediately. This dysfunction responds to specific treatment procedures, and remediation of this disorder will greatly assist Dean to develop his full potential for literacy skills, and a stronger and more flexible vocabulary. He will have difficulty coping with the reading and writing demands of his school curriculum until his auditory system provides him with more adequate sensory information to integrate with the visual units of our alphabet system.
2. When a base of auditory conceptual function has been developed, Dean's independence and self-confidence in transcoding spoken and written language should markedly improve. This, in turn, may ameliorate the attention and concentration problems he has experienced. If it does not, behavior modification is recommended, with the emphasis on the pleasure Dean can take in his ability to monitor and control his attention and concentration.
3. Improved and more stable language comprehension can also be expected to follow on improved auditory conceptual function. If this does not occur spontaneously to the degree expected, visual imagery should be stimulated, as an aid to language comprehension.

Clinician's name, degree, certification
Title

Example of a brief evaluation report following guidelines required by a Health Maintenance Organization (HMO)

August 1, 1986

Re: Taylor, Tina
DOB: 6/14/84
Age: 2 yrs. 1 mos.
Referred by: Paul Black, M.D.
            Pediatrician

Speech and Language Evaluation

Complaint: Dr. Black has observed evidence of slow speech and language development. Parents expressed concern to him and requested evaluation. Little evidence of increased expressive skills during the past six months.

History: Tina Taylor is the only child of John and Barbara Taylor. Parents are concerned because Tina speaks a lot of jargon but says few intelligible words. Mother's first language is Italian and she speaks English with a noticeable accent. Father speaks English only.

Mother reports normal pregnancy and delivery. With the exception of late speech onset, developmental milestones are reported as occurring within appropriate time limits. Tina's hearing has been tested and found within normal limits. No feeding or coordination problems are reported. Tina eats many table foods. She finger feeds and uses a spoon to scoop and eat. She drinks from a cup and takes a bottle twice a day.

Parents report Tina responds to her name and will follow simple directions. She will remove her shoes on command and pulls her own socks off. She likes to play with cubes, babies, and a tricycle.

Summary: Tina presents an age-appropriate appearing 2-year-old. She was alert and cooperative during the evaluation. Parents were present providing instructions, praise, and assistance as needed.

Tina understood the meaning of simple directions and prohibitions. She knew at least 3 body parts. She recognized familiar objects and toys. She imitated simple actions (bye-bye, pattycake). She indicated wants and responses by gestures and occasional vocalizations.

Expressively Tina says less than 10 words (reported). She babbled during play. Tina gestured for many wants and responses. Gesture behavior noted included; nodding, waving, pointing, crying, and using facial gestures. She repeated "oh."

Impressions: Delayed speech development, etiology unknown. Hearing is within normal limits. Receptive language, gross, and fine motor development and social behavior appear age-appropriate.

Recommendations: Six sessions of language facilitation training are recommended for parents. Reevaluation in 9 months.

Goals:
1. Provide parents with language development and facilitation guide *Teach Your Child To Talk: A Parent Guide.*
2. Teach parents to increase Tina's preliminary communication skills and functional play.
3. Improve motor imitation.
4. Teach sound imitation and single words.

Clinician's name, degree, etc.
Title

EVALUATION PROFILE FOR YOUNG STUTTERERS

Kenneth J. Knepflar, Ph.D.

NAME _____ AGE _____

ADDRESS _____

_____ TELEPHONE _____

EVALUATION DATE _____CLINICIAN _____

Age at onset of stuttering _____ Factors related to laterality _____

_____

Prevalence of normal disfluencies_____

_____

Disfluency types_____

_____

Descriptions of early symptoms_____

_____

How family responded_____

Descriptions of current symptoms_____

Family history of stuttering_____

_____

_____

_____

_____

_____

_____

_____

_____

_____

FACTORS RELATED TO SPEECH AND LANGUAGE

____ Delayed speech and language development_____

____ Articulation problem_____

____ Vocal variations_____

____ Delayed or abnormal motor development_____

____ Bilingual influences_____

____ Reading problem_____

FACTORS RELATING TO SPEAKING ENVIRONMENT
____ Parental vocabulary level and linguistic complexity _____

____ Familial speaking rate_____

____ Parental speaking fluency_____

____ Frequent interruptions during conversational attempts_____

____ Kind and amount of speech and language stimulation _____

____ Pressure resulting from speech and language correction by adults or other children

____ Teasing, mimicing, or other negative reactions to disfluencies _____

SOCIAL FACTORS
____ Marital or familial problems _____

____ Lack of patience—expecting the child to function beyond capacity_

____ Frequent negative reactions to child _____

____ Parental compulsivity (neatness, tidiness, excessive politeness) ____

____ Failure to accept child as an individual ("Pouring into a mold") ___

____ Emotional shocks or accidents _____

PERSONALITY TRAITS OF CHILD
____ Compulsivity _____

____ Hypersensitivity _____

____ Impatience _____

____ Unrealistic self expectations _____

____ Other _____

SUMMARY OF SIGNIFICANT FACTORS

_____

_____

_____

_____

FINAL DIAGNOSIS

_____

_____

_____

_____

PROGNOSIS

_____

_____

RECOMMENDATIONS

_____

_____

_____

_____

_____

_____

_____

Note. The significance of causal factors is based on a 5-point scale: (0) not significant, (1) very minor significance, (2) mildly significant, (3) moderately significant, (4) very significant, (5) extremely significant.

EVALUATION FORM FOR LARYNGECTOMIZED PATIENTS

Kenneth J. Knepflar, Ph.D.

Name _____ Age _____ Date _____

Address _____ Telephone _____

Source of Referral _____

Current communication status _____

____ esophageal speech,   ____ pharyngeal speech
____ buccal speech,   ____ artificial larynx
____ pseudowhisper,   ____ other _____

1. *Operative Factors*
   Date(s) of surgery _____
   Extent of surgery _____
   _____
   _____
   Postoperative complications _____
   _____
   Irradiation and other treatment procedures _____
   _____
   _____

2. *Physical Factors*
   General physical condition _____
   _____
   Spread of cancer _____
   _____
   Upper respiratory conditions _____
   _____
   Other physical factors _____
   _____
   _____

3. *Geriatric Factors*_____

4. *Auditory Factors*
   Audiometric results _____
   _____
   _____
   Comments _____
   _____

5. *Emotional Factors*
   Depression _____
   Motivation _____
   Degree of dependency _____
   Acceptance of esophageal speech _____
   _____
   Other personality traits or problems _____
   _____

6. *Social Factors*
   Educational background _____
   Cultural background _____
   Patient's sociability _____
   _____
   Family attitudes _____
   _____

Vocational aspects _____

Living situation _____

7. *Intellectual Factors*

_____

_____

8. *Articulation Factors*
Motor factors _____
Dental factors _____
Accuracy of articulation _____

Foreign accent _____

9. *Language Factors*
Language comprehension _____

Language usage _____

Summary of pertinent factors _____

Apparent prognosis _____

Recommendations _____

Example of a diagnostic report letter

December 26, 1984

Martin Jones, M.D.
555 Los Angeles St.
Los Angeles, CA 90000

Re: Doe, Joan

Dear Dr. Jones:

Mrs. Joan Doe, age 51, was first seen for a speech and language evaluation in Los Angeles Community Hospital on September 9, 1984 where she was hospitalized because of an overdose of barbiturates. At that time she displayed no apparent language disorder, except for problems of immediate and recent memory. She did, however, exhibit symptoms of severe dysphonia, characterized by poor volume, monotonous pitch, and impaired breathing. Vegetative functions (swallowing, coughing, throat clearing, etc.) were also impaired.

Following dismissal from the hospital, the patient was seen for home treatment at the request of her physicians. She was seen initially once a week, and during the past month, treatment was increased to two times a week.

Although the patient was able to achieve adequate vocal loudness during treatment, carryover to conversational speech was poor. Part of this failure may be attributed to Mrs. Doe's memory deficits, which make it difficult for her to remember events from day to day. Also there was no family member at home during the day on a regular basis to help the patient with home treatment assignments.

At the recommendation of her neurologist, Dr. A. Smith, the patient was hospitalized in the rehabilitation unit of Pasadena Medical Center where it is hoped she will benefit from an intensive and coordinated program of physical and occupational therapy, as well as continued speech pathology services. Mrs. Doe's speech pathology treatment program may be reinstated when she returns home. Thank you for referring Mrs. Doe to me.

Yours sincerely,

Clinician's name, degree, etc.
Title

Example of a Consultation Report to a referring speech-language pathologist

CONSULTATION REPORT

Name: Ben Smith   Referred by: Mrs. Judy Jones, Speech Specialist
                                  Sea View School District

Birthdate: June 1, 1973
Age: 11 years, 4 months   Date of Consultation: October 17, 1984

Background Information: Ben was accompanied to the evaluation by his father, Mr. Tom Smith and his school speech specialist, Mrs. Judy Jones. Mr. Smith stated that Ben's voice disorder has been evident since infancy. No normal vocalizations were present during his early development. Copies of medical and speech pathology reports were reviewed, extending back to 1978. A recent report from James O. Evans, M.D., who saw Ben on September 12, 1984 stated:

The vocal cords are of the usual appearance and move well, but approximation on phonation is not held sufficiently long to permit emission of a sustained tone, and there is insufficient airflow from the lungs to produce a loud tone. This is not because of any intrinsic laryngeal disorder but rather because of lack of sufficient breath support. He seems totally unable to control expiration in the manner required for proper tonal production, and herein lies the key to his therapy.

It is apparent that the most recent medical report suggests that Ben currently has a healthy larynx.

Consultation Requests: Mrs. Jones, Ben's school speech specialist requested the consultation because his work in the schools with previous speech specialists had resulted in clinical failure. She requested specific information regarding Ben's speech pathology diagnosis, prognosis, and treatment plan.

Description of Symptoms: Most of Ben's conversational voice is weak in loudness and low in pitch. His vocal quality is extremely breathy, "raspy" and at times, gutteral. His habitual speaking voice is best classified as a strained whisper, rather than true phonation. Marked neck tensions are present during his speaking attempts.

Clinical Observations: Ben's vocal behavior was observed in sitting, standing, and reclining (face up) positions. No evidence of voluntary diaphragmatic action could be observed under any of these circumstances, even after several demonstrations. His respiratory habits during rest and phonation were observed. During rest, he took approximately 30 inhalations per minute involving shoulder elevation and strained movements of the upper rib cage and clavicular areas. Similarly frequent shallow upper chest inhalations were observed during speaking attempts with considerable effort and strain, which is not present during quiet breathing.

Most of Ben's reflexive vocalizations (coughing, throat clearing, grunting, laughing, and crying) have the same strained acoustic characteristics that are present in his habitual speaking voice. True phonation was elicited only during and following periods of laughter which were stimulated by "tickling" of his rib cage and diaphragmatic-abdominal areas. This stimulation resulted in reflexive diaphragmatic action. During these periods Ben sustained clear phonation for a maximum of approximately five seconds and for as many as eight consecutive syllables during counting. His reflexive laughter during the "tickling" sessions was perceived as being within normal range for a boy his age. These vocalizations were much higher in pitch and greater in loudness than his habitual speaking voice. The strained quality was not present and chest resonance was discernible. During this session, Ben was not able to produce these near-normal vocal tones voluntarily without the stimulation provided by "tickling."

Clinical Impressions: Ben appears to exhibit impairment to the diaphragmatic and abdominal musculature, which has probably prevented normal breathing habits since infancy. (Normal children, during the first year of life, experience extensive "rehearsal" in vocalization with depression of the diaphragm and expansion of the rib cage, resulting in approximation of the vocal cords during reflexive vocalization activities.) Apparently Ben never had these kinds of prespeech "rehearsals," and since he began talking, he has reinforced abnormal respiratory habit patterns.

It is probable that most of the muscles required for normal respiration have never been strengthened through normal use and many muscles, with which he has compensated, are overly developed. It is also probable that there has been extensive over-use of the intrinsic and extrinsic muscles of the larynx, with which he has struggled to speak, instead of allowing air to initiate his phonatory attempts.

In addition to the probable neuromuscular basis for Ben's voice disorder, it is apparent that a significant degree of emotional overlay is present, resulting from frustration and feelings of failure in communicative activities. Furthermore, I suspect that he has high aspirations academically and that he has "pushed" too hard to succeed in a number of areas, thus adding tension and additional frustration.

It is impossible at this time to state a realistic prognosis for Ben's eventual complete vocal habilitation because of the severity and complexity of the problem. I believe, however, that with intensive voice habilitation and effective home carry-over programs, the prognosis for some improvement is excellent.

Recommendations: Mrs. Judy Jones has agreed to see Ben for daily voice therapy in the school setting. Recommended goals for Mrs. Jones in working with Ben are:

1. Practice voluntary use of the diaphragm and abdominal muscles during rest. (Fewer and deeper inhalations per minute.)
2. Extensive work with Ben in a reclining (face up) position with stimulation by "tickling," emphasizing prolonged phonation of vowels, rote material, and short phrases.
3. Mirror work so that Ben will become aware of the visual aspects of his problem (neck strain, shoulder elevation, etc.)
4. Encourage Ben to speak at a slower rate.

Both at home and in the classroom, Ben should be encouraged to relax and to enjoy pleasant, free, enjoyable activities with as little strain and pressure as possible.

I would like to see Ben for a second consultation in approximately two months in order to evaluate progress and assist in planning further treatment for him.

When some progress has been made, I suggest that Ben see Dr. Evans for an additional consultation, to provide medical guidance for his long-range treatment program.

Clinician's name and degree,
Speech Pathologist

cc: Mrs. Judy Jones
    James O. Evans, M.D.
    Mr. and Mrs. Tom Smith

Example of reporting test protocol results regarding fluency. (From a speech-language evaluation report concerning a 4-year-old child who stutters.)

Stuttering Prediction Instrument
Riley and Riley (1981)

This test evaluates the severity of the child's stuttering through an assessment of the quantity and quality of stuttering behavior and the child's and parent's reaction to the stuttering reported by the parent and observed in the child's conversational speech. It aids in quantifying severity and predicting chronicity of the stuttering behavior.

Subtest	Rating	Task score
Reactions	parent concern teasing, frustration, word avoidance	7
Part-Word Repetitions	4 or more, moderate tension	5
Prolongations	none	0
Frequency	2–3%	3

TOTAL SCORE: 15
SEVERITY RATING: 14th percentile - mild

Stuttering Severity Instrument
Riley and Riley (1980)

This test evaluates the severity of the child's stuttering through an assessment of the quantity and quality of stuttering behavior and physical concomitants.

Subtest	Rating	Task score
Frequency	2–3%	6
Duration	2–9 secs.	4
Physical concomitants	none	0

TOTAL SCORE: 10
SEVERITY RATING: 14th percentile - mild

DIAGNOSTIC CODES

☐ 388.4 ABNORMAL AUDITORY PERCEPTION
☐ 750.0 ANKYGLOSSIA
☐ 668.2 ANOXIA
☐ 784.3 APHASIA
☐ 784.41 APHONIA
☐ 343 CEREBRAL PALSY
☐ 437.9 CEREBROVASCULAR DISEASE
☐ 749.1 CLEFT LIP
☐ 749.2 CLEFT LIP & PALATE
☐ 749 CLEFT PALATE
☐ 389.0 CONDUCTIVE HEARING LOSS
524.5 DENTOFACIAL FUNCTIONAL ABNORMALITIES
☐ 784.5 DYSARTHRIA
☐ 784.69 APRAXIA

☐ 787.2 DYSPHAGIA
☐ 781.3 DYSPRAXIA
☐ 345 EPILEPSY
☐ 300.9 HEAD INJURY
☐ 784.49 HOARSENESS/HYPERNASALITY/HYPONASALITY
☐ 389.2 MIXED HEARING LOSS
☐ 382.9 OTITIS MEDIA
☐ 389.10 SENSORINEURAL HEARING LOSS
☐ 784.5 SPEECH DISORDER
☐ 478.5 VOCAL CORD NODULES
☐ 478.3 VOCAL CORD PARALYSIS
☐ 478.4 VOCAL CORD POLYPS
☐ 784.40 VOICE DISTURBANCE UNSPECIFIED
☐ 315.31 DEVELOPMENTAL LANGUAGE DISORDER

Example of a portion of a graphic computerized diagnostic summary:

Southern Los Angeles Center for Communication Disorders
Communication Modality Deficit Summary
Developed by Marguerite Orsten, M.S.P.A., C.C.C.
and Mary M. Serafin, M.S., C.C.C.

Test Administered	Test Description	Extremely Severe	Severe	Moderately Severe	Moderate	Mild	WNL
Percentiles		<1 %ile	1–2 %ile	3–7 %ile	8–16 %ile	17–31 %ile	>32 %ile
Standard Deviation		≤−2.5SD	≤−2SD	≤−1.5SD	≤−1SD	>−1SD	≥−.5SD
Standard Score		≤62	63–70	71–77	78–85	86–92	≥93
Scaled Scores		1–2	3	4–5	6–7	8–9	10–21
AUDITORY PROCESSING							
Ages (Moderate)		<3–5	≥3–5	≥3–9	≥4–1	≥4–6	≥5–0
Auditory Attention (Moderate)							
Subj. Obs.	Aud. Atten.				Moderate		
Auditory Acuity (WNL)							
Hgr. Scr.	Hear Screen						WNL
Oral Dis. Seq. & Concpt. (WNL)							
TOLD-PO	Word Discrim					9 SS,	37 %ile
WeissArtic	Aud. Discrim.						WNL
Aud. Short-term Memory (WNL)							
TOLD-P	Sen. Imit.					9 SS,	37 %ile
	Listening						106 SS
Token Test	TT III						>−.5SD
	TT V						>−.5SD
	TT I						w/i +1SD
	TT IV						>−.5SD
	TT II						w/i +1SD
Integrative Processing (WNL)							
TOLD-P	Gram.Undstg.						11 SS, 63 %ile
Token Test	TT V						−.5SD
WRT/Long-term Memory (Mild)							
Sub. Obs.	WRT/Lg.Tm.Mm.				Moderate		

APPENDIX C

PROGRESS NOTES
PROGRESS REPORTS
DISCHARGE SUMMARY

Example of Progress Notes for a 4-year-old boy with delayed speech/language

4/26/88 *Goal:* To improve use of "are" auxiliary in longer sentences contrasted with auxiliary "is."

Used picture cards and then a storybook to elicit productions of auxiliary "/is/" and /are/. Focused on "are" with complex subjects such as the boy and the girl are _____ing in which Charlie typically omits the auxiliary or substitutes "is." When given indirect model during storytelling his accuracy is 55% which increases to 85% with direct model. Future goals are:

1. Continue as above.
2. Introduce possessive pronouns.
3. Introduce auxiliary "am" and include in sentences of increasing length and complex sentences.

4/28/88 *Goal:* Improve use of complex sentences constructs.

Used Concept Lotto to elicit/model sentences with n + goes with + n + and the - is -ing and other targets from past sessions. He was quiet and reticent today because new therapist was in room to observe. He is now using "am" outside of structured activity but does use is "or" consistently.

5/3/88 *Goal:* Improve consistent use of auxiliary "am."

Used Flintstones game and storybook to elicit production of "am." Eighty percent accuracy with direct model and 55% accuracy with indirect model (i.e., during interactive storytelling). Need to continue this and introduce regular past tense (end) and possessive pronouns.

5/5/88 *Goal:* Improve use of auxiliary "am" and subject + is-verbing.

Used Flintstone game and storybook to elicit correct use of "am" + verbing. Direct model "I am" was 80% accuracy, 40% accuracy with modeling/cue of just "I." Continue with correct regular past tense of verb usage also.

Example of Complete Progress Notes for Hospital Patient With Severe Dysarthria

1/8/84

Introduced Proprioceptive Neuromuscular Facilitation (PNF) techniques: 6 icing routines of applied stroking to obicularis oris, buccal area, and posterior tongue to precede other oral exercises. These applications are designed to stimulate oral muscle response, facilitate swallow, and reduce drooling. Worked with basic vowel sounds: /a/, /e/, /i/, /o/, /u/ attempting to increase maximum phonation time. (Maximum on /a/ today 5 sec.) Used mirror to decrease visible evidences of vocal strain. Worked on comfortable diaphragmatic-abdominal breathing during silence and quiet phonation, with slow steady exhalation. Patient was cooperative and enthusiastic. She frequently "tried too hard." Left list of prolonged vowel exercises to be carried out daily.

1/15/84

Added resistance (PNF) technique to increase awareness and strengthen tongue response for elevation and retraction needs. With wooden tongue blade "walked back" on tongue, resisted protrusion, and lateral pushing. Also added tongue and lip suction of the ice pop. Reinforced prolonged phonation on vowel sounds. (Maximum 10 seconds one time but could not repeat more than 7 seconds.) Used mirror during remainder of session to begin work on independent tongue tip elevation for /t/, /d/, /n/, /l/. Combined these sounds with prolonged vowels: /a/, /e/, /i/, /o/, /u/. Used communication board with the entire alphabet to facilitate conversation. Incorporated vowels with /t/, /d/, /n/, /l/ for short conversational phrases, (i.e., *I want water. Don't do that.* Spoke to nursing staff concerning carryover).

1/22/84

Began session with PNF exercises to facilitate oral motility and strength for phoneme production. Today's treatment program reinforced vowel and tongue tip exercises. Emphasized diaphragmatic breathing and increasing "openness" for improved resonance. Conversation was possible with less help from the communication board. Patient pleased by her progress. She has worked well independently this week and with hospital staff members.

1/29/84

Following stimulation of icing and resistance exercises, used amplification today to reinforce patient's ability to monitor her verbal attempts and reinforce improved, less strained voice quality. Maximum phonation: 14 seconds. Used oral reading of newspaper headlines for vowel and conso-nant /t/, /d/, /n/, /l/ carryover. Patient is much more optimistic with regard to her communication skills. Nurses report she is more willing to try to express needs and wants.

PROGRESS REPORT

NAME: Sally Jones   DATE OF EVALUATION: April 24, 1983
BIRTHDATE: June 27, 1979   AGE: 6 years, 2 months
REFERRED BY: Thomas Doe, M.D.

Nature of Problem: Severe speech and language delay caused by profound loss in auditory acuity resulting from meningitis at the age of 6 months.

Background Information: I first saw Sally on April 24, 1983 for an initial evaluation. Sally has been seen by me for three appointments weekly. At the time she was first seen at the chronological age of 3 years, 10 months, Sally was an extremely immature, manipulative child, who did not respond well to limits of any kind. Her only speech was imitative. Her poor attention span and lack of interest in the spoken word made speechreading almost impossible.

Treatment Summary: Sally has been exposed to a multisensory approach to speech and language training. She has become increasingly more motivated to speak and more aware of the language responses of others. Her receptive vocabulary has increased markedly and more intelligible words are being used. Although a large gesture language has developed, more of her gestures are being accompanied now by verbal responses. Since June, 1985 when Sally's family received training in Cued Speech, her awareness of language and her comprehension of the spoken word have shown marked improvement. Her alertness, awareness, and intellectual curiosity indicate a readiness for a structured educational program designed to meet her needs.

Recommendations:
1. Continue individual speech and language training.
2. Enrollment in a school situation with training involving the use of Cued Speech.

Clinician's name and degree,
Speech Pathologist

Example of a progress report concerning an adult with a voice disorder with a complex medical history

PROGRESS REPORT

NAME: Mitchell, Thomas   AGE: 48
REFERRED BY: Charles Karl, M.D.
DATE OF INITIAL EVALUATION: June 2, 1987
DATE OF THIS REPORT: Jan. 4, 1988
DIAGNOSIS: Moderately severe hyperfunctional dysphonia secondary to
          recurring laryngeal granuloma.

Background Information: At the time of his initial voice evaluation in this office on June 2, 1987. Mr. Mitchell had had three previous surgeries for the removal of laryngeal granuloma. At that time, a small fourth granuloma had already begun to appear. Vocal rehabilitation from June through August was aimed at improving vocal efficiency in an attempt to prevent further progression of the existing granuloma and thus prevent the need for a fourth surgical procedure. Finally, when it became evident that a fourth surgery was necessary, treatment was temporarily discontinued, allowing for a period of total vocal rest postsurgically. On October 6, 1987 postsurgical voice therapy was again scheduled for Mr. Mitchell on the recommendation of Dr. Karl. Sessions have been scheduled once weekly during October, November, and December.

Treatment Summary: Mr. Mitchell's voice therapy has included a program of vocal exercises carried out several times daily at home. Treatment goals have included elevation of habitual pitch, expansion of his pitch range, improvement of abdominal breath support for speech, elimination of glottal shock on initial vowels, and increasing mandibular excursion during speech. All treatment procedures have been aimed at preventing a recurrence of Mr. Mitchell's laryngeal granuloma.

Progress Summary: Since his last surgery in September, Mr. Mitchell's progress has been excellent. His breathing habits for speech have improved significantly. Abdominal breath support for speech is now present about 75% of the time. His habitual speaking pitch is also appropriate 75% to 80% of the time. Evidences of vocal misuse are still present under circumstances involving physical fatigue and time pressure.

Several consultations with Dr. Karl have confirmed the fact that Mr. Mitchell's vocal cords continue to be clear, with no evidence of another granuloma.

Recommendations: Mr. Mitchell should continue voice therapy once weekly during the month of January. Then the frequency of treatment sessions will gradually be reduced as progress allows. If no complications arise, it should be possible to discontinue treatment within a 6- to 9-month period.

Example of a Discharge Report concerning a 21-year-old with a severe voice disorder. (Treatment discontinued prematurely.)

DISCHARGE SUMMARY

NAME: Dover, Peter   AGE: 21
REFERRED BY: John M. Homer, M.D.
INITIAL EVALUATION: October 28, 1986
DATE OF THIS REPORT: January 27, 1987
DIAGNOSIS: Severe vocal hyperfunction secondary to postmutational
dysphonia resulting in chronic erythema of the vocal cords.

Treatment Summary: Peter Dover has received a total of 14 individual voice therapy sessions to date. Treatment techniques have included: (a) exercises aimed at the development of diaphragmatic breathing and abdominal breath support, (b) vocal exercises aimed at gradual lowering of the voice, (c) increased maximum phonation time on lower-pitched sounds, (d) increasing vocal loudness in voice exercises and conversation, (e) increasing mandibular excursion during speaking, and (f) eliminating habitual elevation of the larynx during speech attempts.

Voice therapy has been accompanied by relaxation techniques and communication counseling.

Progress Summary: During many of his sessions, Peter was able to produce a lower adult male voice during vowel prolongation and in short phrases. Initial success at lowering the voice was achieved through singing, rather than speaking. During relaxed periods Peter is achieving some success at carrying over new vocal habits outside the therapy setting.

Recommendations: Two treatment sessions per week should continue, but because of financial factors, Mr. and Mrs. Dover temporarily discontinued David's treatment as of January 27, 1987.

Clinician's name, degree, certification
Title(s)

APPENDIX D

STATEMENT CONCERNING PAYMENT FOR
SERVICES RENDERED
SPEECH PATHOLOGY AND AUDIOLOGY PLAN OF
TREATMENT FORM
SPEECH PATHOLOGY CARE PLAN

INSURANCE AND PAYMENT FOR SPEECH PATHOLOGY SERVICES

In order to prevent misunderstanding about medical insurance we wish to point out that:

1. All professional services furnished are charged directly to the patients.

2. Patients are personally responsible for payment of bills.

3. Patients should expect to keep their accounts current while waiting for their insurance company to make payment.

Your insurance coverage is a contract between you and your insurance company to help you meet medical expenses. It is not possible for us to provide service on the basis that the insuror will always pay all charges, as coverage varies so greatly among companies.

We will be glad to prepare the reports necessary to help you collect your benefits from your insurance company.

Should your insuror send us any check we will credit the amount to your account or endorse it to you if your bill is already paid. Please feel free to discuss charges at any time.

EECH PATHOLOGY AND AUDIOLOGY
N OF TREATMENT

1 PERIOD COVERED BY THIS REPORT: ☐ INITIAL ☐ INTERIM ☐ DISCHARGE	**2** DATES OF SERVICE: **3** NO. OF TREATMENTS:

ATIENT'S NAME (LAST, FIRST, INITITAL):   **5** HIC NUMBER OR ID NUMBER: **6** AGE: **7** DATE OF BIRTH:

ROVIDER NAME: **9** PROVIDER NO.:   **10** PLACE OF TREATMENT: ☐ HOME ☐ OFFICE ☐ HOSP. I.P. ☐ HOSP. O.P.

DMITTING DIAGNOSIS: **12** DATE OF ONSET: **13** DATE PLAN ESTAB.:

AST SPEECH PATHOLOGY TREATMENT: **15** INSURANCE COVERAGE:
☐ NO   ☐ YES – DATES (IF KNOWN):   ☐ MEDICARE-A ☐ MEDICARE-B ☐ MEDI-CAL ☐ PRIVATE INS.

PEECH AND LANGUAGE DIAGNOSIS:

TYPE(S), SEVERITY AND PROGNOSIS:

FUNCTIONAL GOALS AND TREATMENT PLAN:

FREQUENCY AND ESTIMATED DURATION OF TREATMENT:

RECOMMENDATIONS (INSTRUCTIONS TO NURSING STAFF AND/OR FAMILY):

UNCTIONAL STATUS REPORT: DEGREE OF IMPAIRMENT   (SEE INSTRUCTIONS ON REVERSE SIDE FOR KEY)

FUNCTION	INIT.	BEGIN OF BILL PERIOD	PRES.	NARRATIVE PROGRESS:
ITORY COMP.				
GUAGE EXPR.				
ECH INTELL.				
AL COMP.				
DING COMP.				
PH. FORM				
THMETIC				
-VERBAL COMM.				
LLOWING				
E				
RING				
ODY				
ENCY RESP.				
FUSION				
ENTION SPAN				
ECTIVE ATTENTION				
ORY				
GHT ORGANIZATION				
GMENT				

EASON FOR DISCHARGE:

PEECH PATHOLOGIST SIGNATURE AND LICENSE NUMBER: **20** DATE:

CERTIFY_____ RE-CERTIFY_____ THAT I HAVE EXAMINED THE PATIENT AND SPEECH PATHOLOGY IS NECESSARY AND THAT SERVICE WILL BE REVIEWED EVERY 30 DAYS

R MORE OFTEN IF THE PATIENT'S CONDITION REQUIRES. I ESTIMATE THAT THESE SERVICES WILL BE NEEDED FOR ABOUT_____

PECIFY NUMBER OF DAYS, WEEKS, OR MONTHS.)*   COMMENTS:

HYSICIAN'S NAME: **23** PHYSICIAN'S SIGNATURE: **24** DATE: **25** TELEPHONE:

11/75   *SEE INSTRUCTIONS FOR PREPARATION ON REVERSE SIDE.   WHITE — PROVIDER; CANARY — FISCAL INTERMEDIARY; PINK — SPEECH PATH. DEPT.; GOLDENROD — PHYSICIAN.

INSTRUCTIONS FOR COMPLETING SPEECH PATHOLOGY PLAN OF TREATMENT INFORMATION FORM

1. Enter an X to indicate an initial, interim or discharge period of service. If form covers both initial and discharge information, check both.
2. Enter the beginning and ending dates of the period covered by this report
3., 4., 5., 6., 7. Record information as indicated.
8. Enter X in appropriate box to show where treatment was provided.
9. Enter information as indicated.
10. Enter the diagnosis of the medical problem.
11. Enter onset date of the medical problem.
12. Enter the month, day and year that the physician first ordered the services to be provided. DO NOT CHANGE THIS DATE ON INTERIM BILLINGS.
13. Enter X in appropriate box. If patient has had prior treatment under a different plan, please indicate dates of prior treatment, if known.
14. Enter X in appropriate box to indicate patient's insurance coverage.
15. Speech and Language Diagnosis.
15A. Type(s)   Refer to speech pathology guidelines. Specify: (1) Which area(s) of general communication abilities are impaired; (2) The primary causal factor(s); and (3) Secondary causal factors if they exist.
     Severity   Refer to the guidelines. Select the descriptive functional impairment term that is most appropriate for each applicable communication category: Extremely Severe, Severe, Moderately Severe, Mild, and Minimal.
     Prognosis   Refer to the guidelines. Indicate the highest level of functional communication the patient will be able to attain. (Community Communicator, Limited Communicator, Assisted Communicator, No Communication Potential.)
15B. Goals and Objectives:
     Goals: A statement of what you intend to help the patient attain by a certain point in time.
     Objectives: A statement that indicates how the patient will benefit from the goals you have set.
15C. Treatment Plan: Describe the treatment approaches that will be utilized in relation to the stated goals and objectives. Include specific procedures, methods and techniques.
15D. Record frequency and estimated duration of treatment necessary to reach stated potential. Refer to the guidelines.
15E. State how the family and/or staff can best communicate with the patient as well as what they should do and/or not do in order to support the patient's treatment program.
16. Functional Status Report
    "Initial" Enter degree of functional impairment (minimal, mild, moderate, moderately severe, and severe) at the time of the initial evaluation.
    "Beginning of This Billing Period" Compare the patient's functional status at the beginning of the billing period with "Initial." Enter in each applicable category: (+) Improved; (√) Remained same; (−) Worse.
    "Present" Compare patient's status from beginning of billing period to end of billing period by indicating: Improved (+); Remained the same (√); or Became worse (−).
    "Narrative Progress" Give a brief description of the changes noted above and their impact on the patient's ability to communicate.
17. Enter the number of treatments given during the period covered by this report.
18. Enter the average length of time of treatment.
19. Complete this section with the final billing.
20., 21. Record therapist's signature and date form was completed.
22. This section can be used as M.D. certification for treatment. If the provider has another means of certifying treatment, the M.D. is not required to sign this form. The Comment Section is an optional area for M.D. to further substantiate need for therapy.
23. Optional.
24., 25. If the form is used as certification of treatment, the M.D. must sign and date this section.
26. Optional.

APPENDIX E

SPECIAL REPORTS AND FORMS
REFERRAL ACKNOWLEDGMENT
INDIVIDUALIZED EDUCATIONAL PLAN (IEP)
SPECIAL REPORTS AND SUMMARIES FOR
TEACHERS OR PARENTS
HEAD START GRANTEE FUNCTIONAL ASSESSMENT FORM
REPORT OUTLINE FOR MEDICAL RECORD
SUPPLEMENTARY INFORMATION FORM

Reevaluation report summary for a Home Health Agency

Mrs. Williams was seen on May 10, 1984 to resume speech pathology services for aphasia following a stroke approximately 3 months ago. The patient had been readmitted to the hospital for head pain. Test results indicate the patient retained recent gains in communication. (See PICA Test results.) Presenting communication problems are in word finding and severe delays in initiating, with verbalizations limited to single words and short phrases. The patient has adequate reading ability and can read orally; handwriting is lost due to right hand paresis. Prognosis appears good to increase conversational adequacy by using oral reading to increase initiation of responses and length of response.

Goals: (a) to reduce time delays, (b) to increase single word and phrase use, (c) to encourage handwriting transition to the left hand.

Treatment Plan: (a) exercises of recognition and recall of symbols, (b) visual and auditory stimulation for single words, phrases, and sentences, (c) digit and phoneme sequencing, (d) instruction of family and Home Health Aide in practice exercises and understanding of patient's limitations and assets, (e) encourage patient to accept deficits and use residual capabilities such as reading; general emotional and supportive activities. It is requested that this patient be seen three times weekly.

Example of a concisely written summary evaluation report written for a patient's hospital ledger (patient was evaluated in an Intensive Care Unit)

Mr. Stanley Smith was seen for speech-language pathology services on May 21, 1984 following a cerebral vascular accident approximately 2 months ago. The patient attended to visual and auditory stimuli and was generally most cooperative during the 40-minute session. Sub-tests of the Porch Index of Communicative Ability, Keenan Aphasia Test, and the

Minnesota Test for Differential Diagnosis of Aphasia were administered. Test results indicate no functional speech. The patient was unable to emit single phonemes such as (a), (i), (u), (e), (ai) or (o). His coughing reaction is extremely weak, and breath pressure for approximating the vocal cords is reduced. He successfully completed the lingua-stabilization test following verbal instruction as opposed to visual imitation. Moderate reduction in oral comprehension of language exists as the length of spoken units are increased. He recognizes common words, discriminates between paired words, recognizes letters and numerals, and numerical concepts are intact. The patient did not read orally. However, reading input was functional for single words, phrases, and short sentences in activities involving matching forms and words to pictures. Gesture and graphic functioning is severely impaired due to weakness and/or paralysis of the upper extremities.

Prognosis: Prognosis is guarded at this time. However, since auditory input is functional to the short sentence level and the patient has age in his favor (only 42), it would appear that communicating needs and wants through a combined nonverbal-verbal (single words, phrases) means may be possible. A 30-day trial period of treatment three times weekly is suggested with further evaluation.

Treatment Plan: Goals: (a) Increase voluntary control of the articulators for phonemic sequencing. (b) Achieve vowels, syllables, and then words. (c) Increase auditory retention. (d) Improve reading skills. (e) Further assess writing potential when the patient is stronger. (f) Instruct other health team members such as nurses, aides, physical therapists, and family to speak slowly, using short sentences with the patient. (g) Muscle strengthening exercises for the tongue and lips. (h) Provide visual and auditory stimulation for words, phrases, and sentences. (i) Have patient listen to his verbal responses and correct his errors. (j) Transfer skills into conversational speech.

Referral Acknowledgment Format

Date _____

THANK YOU _____

for referring _____

Your confidence is appreciated.

Patient was seen on _____

for initial evaluation and a full report will be sent to you upon completion.

Comment: _____

_____

_____

_____

_____

_____

Speech-Language Pathologist

NAME OF PUPIL		BIRTHDATE	DATE	SERVICE PROVIDED BY (USE SOURCE CODE)	PROJECTED DATE OF ACCOMPLISHMENT
	OBJ. NO.	NOTE LEVELS OF EDUCATIONAL PERFORMANCE IN AREAS RELATING TO SPECIAL NEEDS (i.e., ACADEMIC, SOCIAL-ADAPTIVE, PSYCHO-MOTOR, PRE-VOCATIONAL, SELF-HELP, SPEECH/LANGUAGE, INTELLECTUAL, MEDICAL, LSS, NES). SUCH DATA SHOULD INCLUDE STRENGTHS AND NEEDS.	LIST ANNUAL GOALS AND SHORT TERM OBJECTIVES. INCLUDE MEASUREMENT CRITERIA AND RELATE TO PERFORMANCE LEVELS.		
OBJ. REV.	DATE MET				
			GOAL............. OBJECTIVE(S)		
			GOAL............. OBJECTIVE(S)		
			GOAL............. OBJECTIVE(S)		

DIRECTIONS: Under Column 1 headings indicate (1) Examiner/Source*: (2) Assessment Date (where applicable): (3) Data supporting functional descriptions/strengths and needs. Where appropriate, include information from the classroom observation and parent input.

*SOURCE ABBREVIATION CODE:

Pa = Parent	PS = Program Specialist	T = Teacher
A = Administrator	Outside - Agency/Medical Report	Nu = School Nurse
Au = Audiologist	Psyc. = Psychologist	SDi. = District
LSS = Language/Speech Specialist	APE = Adapted Physical Education	

NOTE: A pupil's individual program includes all areas of the curriculum appropriate to his/her level(s) of functioning. The above goals and objectives are written in priority areas of instruction to ameliorate the effects of the handicapping condition(s).

Example of a diagnostic report to a multidisciplinary team mandated by PL 99-457 to assess and serve handicapped and at-risk infants and their families. Information will be used for the Individual Family Service Plan (IFSP) that will be devised by the parents and team.

Carol, an 8-month-old infant with Down syndrome and her parents, John (age 27) and Katie (age 23) Brown, were seen in their home for an infant and family assessment on November 17, 1988. The assessment was done at 5:00 p.m. to accommodate the work schedules of both parents and to observe Carol while she was feeding. Carol is an only child and was delivered after a normal pregnancy (see history in file). The entire assessment was videotaped. The following assessments were completed:

Infant Skills:

Cognitive, fine motor, gross motor, expressive language, social-emotional and self-help were assessed through the Hawaii Early Learning Profile (HELP), a criterion referenced check-list for formulation of intervention goals. Norms were not applied because Carol qualifies for service due to her diagnosis of Down syndrome.

Oral-motor skills were assessed by observing Katie feed Carol. Carol eats table food while sitting in her high-chair with supporting towels around her. She does not take liquids from a cup but uses a bottle, as she has since birth. When the spoon approaches her mouth she leans forward and must raise her hands for balance. A munching pattern, rather than a rotary chew, was noted. She can not bite through a cracker. She exhibited hypotonia of the oral-motor musculature and thrust her tongue out to meet each spoonful. Katie faced Carol and talked to her while feeding.

Interaction: Infant. Some of the Communication Temptations from the Communication Symbolic Behavior Scale were administered to Carol. The clinician opened a jar of bubbles, blew some bubbles, then closed the jar and handed it to Carol. Carol put the jar to her mouth and held it in both hands but did not seek help from one of the adults present. When the clinician ate a cracker in front of her without offering any to her, she made no effort to get the cracker.

Hearing: Hearing will be assessed in the clinic on December 2, 1988. She has had two ear infections. The last one was two months ago.

Interaction: Parent.

The Observation of Communicative Interaction, a check-list to record the mother's behaviors in interaction was filled out from the videotape. Katie was asked to play on the floor with Carol as she usually did. Katie was noted to provide appropriate tactile and kinesthetic stimulation through patting and cuddling Carol. She positioned Carol so that they had eye contact. She was not noted to encourage "conversation," to respond contingently to Carol's behavior or to modify her behavior in response to negative cues from Carol.

Family Assessment:

The Family Needs Survey, a checklist of parent perception of needs, was administered to John and Katie simultaneously and without conversation between them. They were each asked to write down the five most pressing needs for their family. The survey was then discussed with them. Family strengths were thought to be their secure financial situation, their family functioning (they are supportive of each other) and their extended families. Areas of need that they both identified were need for information about Carol's condition, what to expect in the future, and need to assess community resources. Katie identified a need for accepting Carol's condition and John needed more opportunity to meet and talk to other parents of handicapped children. They have not received genetics counseling nor do they belong to a support group.

Conclusions:

Carol's cognitive, fine-motor, gross-motor, expressive language, social-emotional, and self-help skills are slightly delayed, commensurate with Down syndrome. Her family has a number of strengths in that they are supportive of each other and do not need financial aid at this time for Carol's special needs. The parents agree with the clinician's assessment of their needs: information and access to community resources, including genetics counseling, and a parent support group. Services to this family should include: (a) a home visit once per week for parents and Carol; (b) a team approach to accessing community resources including the genetics clinic and the Down Parents Support Group; (c) intervention to focus on Carol's interaction with both parents while playing and feeding; and (d) work with the parents on oral-motor activities for Carol.

Excerpt from a report of a 4-year-old Chinese-American boy with limited English proficiency (LEP)

Note: Space limitations prevented the complete reproduction of the following report in this text. Preceding the portions printed here were sections including developmental history, medical history, speech and language development, family history, educational history, prior evaluations and speech-language services and the clinical assessment of behavior.

HEAD START GRANTEE
FUNCTIONAL ASSESSMENT

NAME OF CHILD (LAST)	(FIRST)	(MIDDLE)	BIRTHDATE (MONTH/DAY/YEAR)
Mendosa	Carlos		09/21/87

HEAD START AGENCY

In order to develop an Individualized Educational Plan (IEP) for the above named child, a comprehensive response to the following is needed.

SECTION I—FUNCTIONAL DESCRIPTION(S)

a. Description(s) of problems and needs _____

Carlos is an attentive and cooperative child who speaks both English and
Spanish. Testing reveals that he is omitting grammatical components of words
which indicate plurals, tenses, and comparatives. He is also omitting sounds
during conversational speech which makes it difficult to understand him at times.

b. Description(s) of strengths

attentive and has age appropriate vocabulary.

SECTION II—RECOMMENDATIONS

a. Provide *specific* recommendations for program services including *special* equipment or materials, instructional/therapeutic services, etc.

speech (1) Carlos will use 5 word sentences incorporating the past, present and
future tenses

teacher (1) stress the concepts of yesterday, today and tomorrow so that Rudolfo
is more aware of time differences

b. Restrictions

none/ can speak both English and Spanish

SECTION III—ASSESSMENT PROCEDURES

ASSESSMENT INSTRUMENTS/METHODS EMPLOYED	DATE
PPVT/Span/Eng.	
ZPLS/Span/Eng.	
Teacher interview	
spontaneous language sample/artic testing	

PLEASE RETURN COMPLETED FORM TO:

NAME	AGENCY	
ADDRESS	CITY	ZIP CODE

Language and Communication Skills:

Formal assessment of language comprehension and language production was not possible due to W.Y.'s lack of attention and unwillingness to do the tasks. Informal assessments revealed the following:

1. *Overall Communication Style*: W.Y. showed a general lack of attention for structured tasks attempted. This included activities that required him to sit down at a table and work quietly. W.Y. was easily distracted by other objects in the environment such as the light on the ceiling, the chair in the corner, etc. His attention span was approximately 3 to 4 minutes long. There was a general lack of response to questions and inadequate turn taking skills exhibited during conversation. When questions were asked, W.Y. would not consistently respond.

2. *Overall Comprehension*: Screening for comprehension was attempted with the Preschool Language Scale (Zimmerman, 1980). W.Y. was not able to attend to this test for longer than 2 minutes. Therefore, a precise indication of his language comprehension in English was not obtained. Informal assessment indicated that W.Y. was able to understand simple one stage commands and some two stage commands—"close the door," "take the car and put it on the table"—both in Mandarin Chinese and in English. The lack of response to questions may be a function of not understanding the question or possibly an unwillingness to answer. In certain motivating situations W.Y. answered appropriately. For example, to "What did you just do?" he replied, "Step in water." At other times. W.Y. answered with statements that seemingly had no relation to the question being asked. For example, when asked "Who shall I throw it to?" (asked by the clinician who was holding a ball) he replied, "Yah." Although W.Y. seemed to comprehend what was being said to him most of the time, he was inconsistent in responding and frequently unwilling to participate.

3. *Overall Production and Response Pattern*: W.Y.'s speech consists of echolalic responses and ritualized speech. Approximately 30% of his utterances were echolalic (e.g., "Okay, put the car away.") Other utterances included ritualized speech patterns that were successively repeated (e.g., "Go outside, go potty, take a walk, broken.") These repetitions made up about 50% of W.Y.'s language production. Gestures were used instead of words on several occasions to convey wants and needs. Single word utterances were noted when pointing out items or events in the immediate environment—"look teeth, take off." As noted previously, some situations created more appropriate language output than others such as "Step in water." However, this did not occur in the majority of his responses. His response patterns in Mandarin Chinese were very similar to those in English.

4. *Overall Intelligibility*: The English version of the assessment of phonological processes screening test was administered. The following errors were noted: /b/ for /v/ and /w/ for /r/ and /l/. W.Y. was estimated to be 70% intelligible for known context and approximately 50% intelligible for unknown contexts. A screening for Mandarin Chinese was also conducted. W.Y. had difficulty producing the /z/ and the "la."

5. *Overall Affect and Interpersonal Skills*: W.Y. was pleasant and bright throughout most of the test session. Although he became manipulative at times as previously noted, he used eye contact and facial expressions to achieve communicative intent in an effective way. He was not selective with regard to showing affection to strangers. This behavior was interpreted as inappropriate to the situations presented.

6. *Oral Motor*: An oral motor examination was not performed because W.Y. was unwilling to cooperate. However, it was noted that his upper front teeth appear to be pointed. In addition, there were large spaces between the teeth (e.g., diastema).

7. *Voice and Fluency*: W.Y.'s voice was noticeably hoarse and somewhat raspy. This factor contributed to decreased speech intelligibility. Fluency appeared to be within normal limits.

8. *Cognitive Skills*: A thorough cognitive assessment was not obtainable during the testing session. Informal tests were attempted to screen for some cognitive abilities. Object permanence was apparent when objects were hidden from view. The child located these items with no difficulty. Blocks of different sizes were used for a sorting test. W.Y. was unable to sort the blocks by shape, size, or color. W.Y.'s motor development appeared to be below normal. Gross motor abilities were assessed with the Denver Developmental Screening Test. He exhibits gross motor abilities equivalent to about 3 years of age. He was unable to balance on one foot or hop on one foot; it was not clear whether he did not want to do these activities or whether he was unable to do them. Fine motor abilities also appeared to be below normal age level. W.Y. could not copy a circle, a cross, or create a stack of four to six blocks.

9. *Auditory Acuity*: A hearing screening was attempted but could not be completed because of W.Y.'s inattention and lack of cooperation.

Summary:

W.Y. exhibits severe delayed speech and language skills both in his native language and in English. His language production and language comprehension were significantly below age level. An informal assessment of language production revealed the use of ritualized speech, echolalic phrases, and a few meaningful words and phases. Speech intelligibility was decreased due to substitution of certain phonemes in English such as b/v, w/l, and in Mandarin w for r and l and difficulty with /z/.

W.Y.'s language comprehension appeared to be better than his production, although normal testing was not possible. These speech and language difficulties also appear to carryover into Mandarin Chinese, as reported by the mother and also assessed by the Mandarin speaking clinician. Motor skills were judged to be below normal age level as exhibited by W.Y.'s inability to perform age level activities in both gross and fine motor tests. An accurate assessment of W.Y.'s cognitive functioning, auditory acuity, and oral motor mechanism was not possible due to his lack of attention, lack of cooperation, and general behavioral characteristics.

Recommendations:

Recommendations are as follows:
1. Speech/language intervention.
   a. To increase language production to age level in both Mandarin and English.
   b. To increase language comprehension to age level in both Mandarin and English.
   c. To increase attention and decrease impulsivity.
   d. To improve interpersonal skills.
   e. To develop preacademic skills.
   f. To improve articulation of v, r, and l in English, and z and l in Mandarin Chinese.
2. A thorough pediatric neurological examination.
3. A thorough audiological examination.
4. Counseling for parents for behavior management and support.
5. Cognitive assessment for school placement.

Disposition:

At the parent conference the mother expressed interest in enrolling W.Y. in speech and language intervention at this clinic. Other recommendations will be implemented by the parents before February 1988, at which time W.Y. will be starting his speech and language intervention. No interpreters were used for the parent conference because the parents knew sufficient English.

Note: The Chinese speech and language clinician served as the facilitator. When concepts were not clearly explained in English, then Mandarin Chinese was used as the way of explaining the situation. The above case study is an example of the use of informal observations in the assessment of a bilingual Mandarin-English speaking child.

Suggested report outline to enter in patient's chart in skilled nursing facility or hospital

Speech Language
Eval☐ Re-Eval☐

Tests Administered:

Results:

Impressions:

Recommendations:

SUPPLEMENTARY INFORMATION FORM

NAME OF PATIENT _____

SOURCE OF INFORMATION: _____ CONFERENCE,

_____ OBSERVATION, _____ TELEPHONE,

_____ OTHER _____

NAME(S) OF INFORMANT(S) _____

DATE _____ TIME _____

PERSON RECORDING INFORMATION _____

SUMMARY:

COMMENTS:

NSSLHA Publications

The *NSSLHA Journal* and *Clinical Series* are published by the National Student Speech Language Hearing Association. The *NSSLHA Journal* features student-authored reports and papers by selected professionals and members of ASHA whose areas of expertise are considered pertinent to student interests.

NSSLHA Journal (ISSN 0736-0312)

Published annually since 1973. Volumes 15, 16 (1987-1988), each $6.00
Single copies volumes 1-10, each $1.50; Set, $10 plus $1.00 postage and handling; volumes 11-14, each $4.00

Clinical Series (ISSN 0887-6584)

No. 1 *The Parent Interview: Guidelines for Student and Practicing Speech Clinicians,* by Lon Emerick (1969) 1.50

No. 2 *Private Practice: Guidelines for Speech Pathology and Audiology,* edited by Donna R. Fox (1971) 1.50

No. 3 *Instrumentation in the Speech Clinic: A Handbook for Clinicians and Students,* by William Dawson (1973) 1.50

No. 4 *Report Writing in the Field of Communication Disorders: A Handbook for Students and Clinicians* (2nd ed.) by Kenneth J. Knepflar and Annette A. May 7.00

No. 5 *Clinical Oral Language Sampling: A Handbook for Students and Clinicians,* by Sandie Barrie-Blackley, Caroline Ramsey Musselwhite, Stephania Harder Rogister, edited by Sophia Hadjian (1977) 3.95

No. 6 *Report Writing in Audiology,* by Bradley Billings, Henry Schmitz, edited by Dean C. Garstecki (1979) 3.95

No. 7 *Alternate Methods of Communication,* by Faith Carlson, edited by Richard A. Forcucci (1981) 3.95

No. 8 *Pragmaticism: Treatment for Language Disorders,* by Ellen Lucas Arwood, edited by David J. Draper (1983) 4.00

No. 9 *Counseling in Speech and Hearing Practice,* by Robert L. Schum, edited by Eugene B. Cooper (1986) 4.00

No. 10 *Self-Supervision: A Career Tool for Audiologists and Speech-Language Pathologists,* by Patricia L. Casey, Kathryn J. Smith, and Sandra R. Ulrich; edited by Leah C. Lorendo (1988) 6.00

All orders must be prepaid. Credit card charges accepted for orders of $25.00 or more. All publications are available from **Publication Sales, American Speech-Language-Hearing Association, 10801 Rockville Pike, Rockville, MD 20852.**